Life after Cancer in Adoles and Young Adulthood

Adolescence and young adulthood is often a difficult enough time without serious illness. However, research has shown that cancer, and surviving cancer, at this age presents distinctive problems medically, socially and psychologically. This important work offers a glimpse into a previously under-researched area and contributes to a better understanding of the needs of adolescents and young adults post cancer.

Focusing not only on the physical effects, but also the social, cognitive, emotional and physiological consequences of surviving cancer in adolescence and young adulthood, Anne Grinyer draws directly upon data collected from adolescents and young adults who have been treated for cancer. The book is structured around themes they raised such as fertility, life plans, identity, psychological effects and physical effects. These issues are drawn together in the final chapter and related to clinical and professional practice as well as current policy.

This book presents the voices of those who have lived through the experience of cancer in adolescence and young adulthood, and links them to the relevant theoretical and analytical literature. It will be of interest to professionals and researchers in nursing, social work, counselling and medicine as well as medical sociologists, young adults living with cancer and survivors of young adult cancer.

Anne Grinyer is Senior Lecturer in Health Research at Lancaster University, UK.

Life after Cancer in Adolescence and Young Adulthood

The experience of survivorship

Anne Grinyer

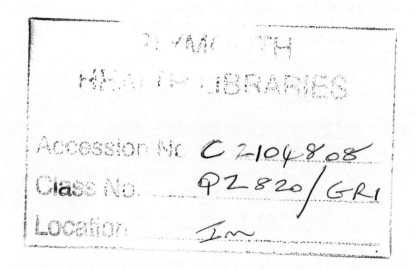
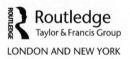

Routledge
Taylor & Francis Group

LONDON AND NEW YORK

First published 2009
by Routledge
2 Park Square, Milton Park, Abingdon, Oxon OX14 4RN

Simultaneously published in the USA and Canada
by Routledge
270 Madison Avenue, New York, NY 10016

*Routledge is an imprint of the Taylor & Francis Group,
an informa business*

© 2009 Anne Grinyer

Typeset in Sabon by Swales & Willis Ltd, Exeter, Devon
Printed and bound in Great Britain by CPI Antony Rowe,
Chippenham, Wiltshire

Library of Congress Cataloging in Publication Data
Grinyer, Anne, 1950–
    Life after cancer in adolescence and young adulthood:
    the experience of survivorship/Anne Grinyer.
    p. cm.
    1. Cancer in adolescence. I. Title.
    [DNLM: 1. Adolescent. 2. Adult. 3. Life Change Events.
    4. Neoplasms—psychology. 5. Survivors. QZ 275 G868L 2009]
    RC281.C4G773 2009
    616.99'400835—dc22
    2008045332

ISBN10: 0–415–47702–6 (hbk)
ISBN10: 0–415–47703–4 (pbk)
ISBN10: 0–203–87880–9 (ebk)

ISBN13: 978–0–415–47702–4 (hbk)
ISBN13: 978–0–415–47703–1 (pbk)
ISBN13: 978–0–203–87880–4 (ebk)

This book is dedicated to the memory of George whose life, illness and death have inspired the last 9 years of my research, and to his parents Helen and Geoff whose support has contributed so much to the understanding and knowledge of the life stage effects of cancer in adolescence and young adulthood. The book is also dedicated to all the participants who shared their stories with me and spoke with such bravery and fortitude of the many challenges they faced in their lives as survivors of young adult cancer.

'… if I had been ten years older then I would have had that bit of my life without interruption.'

(Thomas: 13 years after he was diagnosed with
a brain tumour at the age of 17)

Contents

Acknowledgements

This book could not have been written without the help, support and input of many others. My thanks go to those long-suffering friends and colleagues who read and commented so helpfully on early drafts, they include: Helen, Geoff, Judith, Jennifer, Julie and Jane. The research could not have been conducted without the financial support of the George Easton Memorial Trust and all those who contribute to it. The technical help from Anthony has been invaluable as has the knowledge that I could rely on my stalwart transcriber Karen. I would also like to thank those health professionals who allowed me access to their patients and ex patients. In addition, I owe a huge debt of gratitude to the Lymphoma Association and the Teenage Cancer Trust; both organisations helped me to recruit and provided an invaluable route through which to reach long-term survivors. However, my biggest thanks must go to the participants – those long-term survivors who were willing to share their experiences with me and who trusted me with their life stories. I hope that they will think I have done justice to the material they so generously contributed.

Participants

Survivors

Andrea: Diagnosed at 18 with acute myeloid leukaemia, 39 when interviewed.

Ashley: Diagnosed at 17 with cutaneous T-Cell lymphoma, 54 when interviewed.

Ben: Diagnosed at 18 with testicular cancer, 22 when interviewed.

Bob: Diagnosed at 14 with non-Hodgkin's lymphoma, 62 when interviewed.

Dan: Diagnosed at 21 with testicular cancer, 26 when interviewed.

Debbie: Diagnosed at 24 with Hodgkin's lymphoma, 46 when interviewed.

Elaine: Diagnosed at 21 with Hodgkin's lymphoma, 26 when interviewed.

Elaine B: Diagnosed at 23 with Hodgkin's lymphoma and at 25 with non-Hodgkin's lymphoma, 38 when interviewed.

Gillian: Diagnosed at 20 with Hodgkin's lymphoma, 54 when interviewed.

Greg: Diagnosed at 12 with osteosarcoma, 31 when interviewed.

Helen: Diagnosed at 17 with Hodgkin's lymphoma, 35 when interviewed.

Huxley: Diagnosed at 17 with acute lymphoblastic leukaemia, 35 when interviewed.

Jack: Diagnosed at 14 with Hodgkin's lymphoma, 23 when interviewed.

Jamie: Diagnosed at 21 with testicular cancer, 23 when interviewed.[1]

Janet: Diagnosed at 18 with Hodgkin's lymphoma, 45 when interviewed.

John: Diagnosed at 18 with Hodgkin's lymphoma, 51 when interviewed.

Julie: Diagnosed at 24 with Hodgkin's lymphoma and breast cancer 14 years later, 39 when interviewed.

Kate: Diagnosed at 22 with Hodgkin's lymphoma, 53 when interviewed.

Katie: Diagnosed at 19 with ovarian cancer, 32 when interviewed.

Kelly: Diagnosed at 18 with non-Hodgkin's lymphoma, 25 when interviewed.

Kirsty: Diagnosed at 18 with Hodgkin's lymphoma, 23 when interviewed.

Kristin: Diagnosed at 17 with testicular cancer, 21 when interviewed.

Lesley: Diagnosed at 24 with Hodgkin's lymphoma, 42 when interviewed.

Linda: Diagnosed at 16 with Hodgkin's lymphoma, 44 when interviewed.

Lisa: Diagnosed at 26 with non-Hodgkin's lymphoma, 35 when interviewed.

Louise: Diagnosed at 19 with Ewing's sarcoma, 27 when interviewed.

Majad: Diagnosed at 22 with testicular cancer, 29 when interviewed.

Marc: Diagnosed at 17 with osteosarcoma, 38 when interviewed.

Mary: Diagnosed at 17 with Hodgkin's lymphoma, 41 when interviewed.

Maz: Diagnosed at 24 with Ewing's sarcoma, 28 when interviewed.

Meg: Diagnosed at 20 with Hodgkin's lymphoma, 58 when interviewed.

Michael: Diagnosed at 25 with testicular cancer, 30 when interviewed.

Paul: Diagnosed at 18 with testicular cancer, 27 when interviewed.

Paul B: Diagnosed at 19 with non-Hodgkin's lymphoma, 30 when interviewed.

Phoebe: Diagnosed at 22 with acinic cell carcinoma, 24 when interviewed.[2]

Quentin: Diagnosed at 19 with Hodgkin's lymphoma, 52 when interviewed.

Richard: Diagnosed at 18 with aggressive fibro sarcoma, 54 when interviewed.

Rowena: Diagnosed at 25 with Hodgkin's lymphoma, and with leukaemia 4 years later, 37 when interviewed.

Ruth: Diagnosed at 14 with anaplastic large cell lymphoma, 20 when interviewed.

Scott: Diagnosed at 19 with acute lymphatic leukaemia, 37 when interviewed.

Thomas: Diagnosed at 17 with a brain tumour, 30 when interviewed.

Trevor: Diagnosed at 15 with Hodgkin's lymphoma, 39 when interviewed.

Vicky: Diagnosed at 24 with ovarian cancer, 29 when interviewed.

Family

Anne: Mother of Ruth diagnosed at 14 with anaplastic large cell lymphoma. Ruth was 19 when her mother was interviewed.

Rizwana: Wife of Majad diagnosed at 22 with testicular cancer.

Professionals

Alison: Lead cancer nurse.

Carol: Macmillan nurse.

1 The late effects and long-term consequences of survivorship

My last book based on research with young adults with cancer ended with a question about what happens next. Wolff (2007) claims that while cancer survivorship is increasing, inadequate resources result in the needs of survivors remaining largely unmet by health care providers, yet these needs may be many and varied. As Parsonnet says:

> Adjustment to 'life after cancer' includes the adjustment to physical, emotional, cognitive, social, sexual and spiritual changes, many of which are unforeseen by individuals navigating the worlds of diagnosis and treatment. Late effects vary widely; some are determined by the specific cancer diagnosis and treatment, while others are more dependent upon demographic, personal or social characteristics.
>
> (2007: 2)

Similarly, Stovall (2007) notes that the extent to which a survivor's life is affected in the longer-term is dependent upon a number of variables that include family and cultural relationships, religious beliefs, the treatment received and the progression or resolution of the illness. However, two variables missing from both Stovall and Parsonnet's (2007) observations are age and life stage. I have argued that cancer is both medically and experientially distinct in adolescence and young adulthood[3] (Grinyer 2002a, 2007) thus all those challenges of survivorship raised by Parsonnet (2007) are likely to be exacerbated in this age group. According to Soliman and Agresta (2008) cancer in this age group is unique as it complicates the lives of young people at a period of constant change and as Levitt and Eshelman (2008) point out, the age at diagnosis will result in different fears, needs and requirements for information.[4]

During adolescence and young adulthood a cancer diagnosis will have profoundly disrupted the normal developmental trajectory and this is therefore likely to lead to specific effects on survivorship. It has also been established by Mor *et al.* (1994) that the psychosocial impact of cancer on younger patients is qualitatively different. Older patients may have fewer competing demands on their time and resources and their different expectations may mitigate the negative impact.

Adolescence and young adulthood is a transitional time of life when crucial decisions are made that shape a person's future. It is also a time of turbulence and renegotiation when identities are being formed (Apter 2001). As a result the diagnosis of life-threatening illness may disrupt the life trajectory at a critical moment that can have long-lasting consequences that manifest differently than for other age groups.

As Neville says:

> The survivor of teenage cancer faces many difficulties superimposed on the challenges of a normally tumultuous adolescent life. While research has described the *long-term* effect of teenage cancer on young adulthood, as survivors age, further enquiry into later stages of life is warranted.
>
> (2007: 5, original emphasis)

Langeveld and Arbuckle (2008) say the period after treatment has finished can present additional anxieties as the reality of the situation becomes clear in the post-treatment phase. The longer-term consequences such as the impact on fertility and mortality may not have been processed during treatment and the loss of the relative security of the medical system that once enveloped them may have left the young survivor feeling insecure and unsupported. However, it is not only the psychosocial and emotional outcomes that differ in survivors of adolescent cancer; the aetiology may also be dissimilar to survivors in other age groups (Birch 2005).

So, do the life stage effects of adolescent and young adult cancers continue to shape their survivorship in the longer-term or are the effects mitigated by time? Levitt and Eshelman cite an American epidemiological study that has 'provided volumes of data' (2008: 169) on late effects. While they acknowledge that the results can be extrapolated in some circumstances to include the survivors of adolescent and young adult cancers they claim, like Neville (2007), that more data on this specific population are needed to understand how the life stage of adolescence affects survivorship and, by extension, to answer questions such as: What kind of support is needed after treatment is over? What does survivorship mean for an adolescent or a young adult who has been treated for a life-threatening illness? What are the long-term psychological and emotional consequences? How can the adolescent and young adult be prepared best to manage the challenges that will face them in their future?

The need for research on survivorship was articulated by staff with whom I worked during the research with their adolescent and young adult patients who were still in treatment. The health care workers expressed concerns about the long-term consequences that their patients may have little understanding of and for which they may be unprepared. Indeed, although the last phase of my research was primarily with adolescents and young adults receiving treatment at the time of participation, it also included a few young people not long out of treatment and there were indications from them that a level of ongoing anxiety had been generated by the illness. Gemma feared that every time she had a cold or sore throat it could herald a recurrence and Steven described how he would unthinkingly keep putting his hand on his neck checking for lumps while watching the television (Grinyer 2007).

Survivorship must be the goal of treatment and in no sense do I wish to pathologise survivors many of whom lead healthy and productive lives after their cancers. Nevertheless, questions – not only about the character and quality of that survivorship, but also of how the adolescents and young adults should be prepared for it – arose when talking to those involved in their long-term care. Alison, asked the following questions:

> Is there anything we can do to help? Should there be some mechanism in place for health professionals or other support services to address these issues [such as] further malignancies. You know it is not at all uncommon for people to get second malignancies. I recently was talking to a young girl who was diagnosed with leukaemia at 14 or 15, who in her mid twenties got breast cancer ... she had very high-dose chemotherapy and she had total body radiation, so the chances are this is a result [as] radiotherapy is carcinogenic itself so there's always an increased risk of getting a further malignancy. Whether, if we gave people this information, would it make them unable to live their future lives in a normal way I don't know. I can't, because I've never really discussed it with survivors. I don't know the answers to the questions. And whether, whether they could tell you, I don't know. But I do think it's something that we need to look at and need to explore.
>
> (Alison: lead cancer nurse)

Alison continued by saying that it would be helpful to chart the kinds of challenges that the survivors experience long term in order to prepare them. For example, to develop cognitive problems without knowing why could be extremely distressing. Alison also mentioned that marital breakdown amongst long-term survivors appeared to occur frequently, but whether this was causally related to the illness remained unclear. Alison remembered a surviving patient who had got a first class degree but who could not find a job and others who had got jobs but who, as a direct result of the illness, had failed to get a mortgage or insurance despite a good salary. While Alison acknowledged that giving information to prepare young people for the multiplicity of long-term effects might be desirable, she added that 'currently, as far as we know, that information is not available ... so we cannot point somebody in the [right] direction, even if they want to know.'

So we can see that previous work in the area of teenage cancers has identified that the age and life stage of adolescence and young adulthood (15–25) presents distinct problems (Eden 2006, Grinyer 2007, 2002a, Grinyer and Thomas 2001, Morgan and Hubber 2004) but that while there is a suspicion that the life stage effect will continue to impact on survivorship there is little systematic data to reinforce this informal observation. My central question is, therefore: 'how is long-term survivorship experienced after adolescent and young adult cancer?' Through asking this question of long-term survivors, the issue of whether the life stage effects at diagnosis and treatment persist through survivorship, should become clearer.

However, there is a problem of definition – when does childhood end and adolescence begin and when does young adulthood end and when is maturity reached? The answers to these questions may differ medically and socially and between individual patients, thus drawing firm boundaries presents problems, yet some definition has to be reached. So, for the purposes of this research my definition of a young adult cancer patient is someone diagnosed with and treated for cancer between the ages of 14 and 25.

A working definition of survivorship also needs to be reached. That offered by the National Coalition for Cancer Survivorship is: 'From the time of discovery and for the balance of life, an individual diagnosed with cancer is a survivor' (in Keene *et al.* 2000: 1). Little *et al.* offer the following classification:

> Oncologists count survival as beginning at the time of diagnosis for the purposes of calculating statistics. To them survival means something like 'living at time x', and the survival can then be 'disease-free' or 'with recurrence' ... Some support groups insist that everyone living after a cancer diagnosis is a survivor.
>
> (2000: 501)

Aziz (2007) cites Mullan's interpretation of survivorship which likens the stages to the seasons of the year: 'acute' being the initial stages of diagnosis through to the end of treatment; 'extended' being the post-treatment remission period dominated by regular follow-up and possible intermittent treatment, and finally 'permanent survival', which does not occur at a single moment but which evolves from an extended period of disease-free survival. Aziz (2007) defines long-term survival as 5 or more years beyond the diagnosis of the primary disease.

However, 'survivors' themselves use their own definitions, for example one of four 'survivors' speaking at a conference on Teenage and Young Adult Cancer Medicine said 'I'm not a survivor, I'm just me' (*Contact* 2007: 5). While survivorship may well begin at diagnosis, this study is on late effects and long-term consequences, thus for the purpose of this research I have recruited survivors who are more than four years out of the treatment period.

Some definition of late effects also needs to be reached. According to Levitt and Eshelman: Late effects are defined as the physical, psychological, social and/or economic chronic or late occurring consequences of cancer treatment persisting or occurring at least 5 years from diagnosis (2008: 169).

These authors continue by pointing out that clinically relevant morbidity can vary from that evident at the end of treatment to sequelae that do not manifest until many years later. My participants range in time since diagnosis from four years, to more than 40 years, thus allowing us to enquire into the later stages of life specified as necessary by Neville (2007).

However, there is a distinction between late effects and long-term effects. Aziz defines late effects as 'unrecognised toxicities that are absent or subclinical at the end of therapy and become manifest later', while he says that long-term effects 'refer to any side effects or complications of the treatment for which a cancer patient must compensate' (2007: 55). Long-term effects may also be regarded as 'persistent' in that they begin during the treatment phase and continue beyond it while late effects, in contrast, appear months or years after the completion of treatment. However, Aziz continues by saying that even amongst experts there is disagreement about whether cognitive problems, fatigue, lymphoedema and peripheral neuropathy are late effects or long-term effects. However, my participants tended not to make such distinctions when discussing the long-term/late effects they experience, thus I use their definitions rather than a strictly clinical classification of the longer-term impacts.

That survivorship in this age group is a concern is evidenced by a special 'Survivors' issue of the publication *Contact* (2007), a magazine devoted to issues relating to cancer in children and young people. In this edition young people address the issues that are important to them such as the sadness felt for the friends who did not survive, and the concomitant burden to do well. As one young woman, Clare, said 'The main guilt comes on what for many of us would be a normal bad day and remembering those who do not experience them. It is horrendous to see people dying, there is pressure to do well, be positive at all times, at times that pressure can drive you mad' (2007: 5). However, survivorship was not the main identity of the young people whose other achievements outweighed those of surviving their cancer with the implication that they did not want to become 'professional survivors'.

In the same edition of *Contact* Sophie Broere says the following about her diagnosis at 17 with Hodgkin's lymphoma.

> After a few years, once I felt physically strong and able to trust my body again, I was able to deal with the suppressed emotions resulting from my experience. I cried, and allowed myself to be angry for the first time. Before then I had always felt that I had to be happy and positive, but underlying this, there was a lot of sadness, which I did not want to deal with, as I was afraid of the powerful emotions it might bring out.
>
> (2007: 10)

This contribution echoes Clare's about the pressure to be positive, whether this and Sophie's suppressed emotions would have been experienced in the same way had she been diagnosed during earlier childhood is unclear, but given what we know about developmental issues and the psychology of adolescence it seems that a younger child may be left with a different emotional legacy (Grinyer 2002, 2007).

Alison, lead cancer nurse, suggested that viewing the ongoing emotional effects as 'Post Traumatic Stress' (PTS) might be a useful way to interpret the survivors' experiences. Clearly any measure that limits, or identifies and manages PTS effectively, would have longer-term benefits.

While we know that some adolescent and young adult cancers and or their treatments can lead to secondary cancer or treatment-related cancer in later life, it seems that the experience of having cancer a second time is worse because of the earlier illness. In an interview with Carol, a Macmillan nurse, she said the following when talking about a man in his 40s who developed another treatment-related cancer:

> They think that the tonsil cancer was caused by the treatment that he had for his testicular cancer and that it wasn't a secondary ... now he was 40 he still found it hard to talk about how he was feeling ... it brought back all of how he'd felt, that sense of kind of helplessness and fear. He told me it just made him feel just as he did when he was a young man ... They do react differently [to having it a second time] , definitely ... I can draw on the experience of some of the women who I've met with breast cancer, having had treatment for Hodgkin's as young adults. They feel that life's dealt them a really hard blow ... they say it's not fair they've already had treatment, it's not fair ... why is this happening again?
>
> (Carol: Macmillan nurse)

This of course also raises the question of how and when adolescent and young adult cancer patients should be warned about late effects. But even without any prior warning cancer survivors can interpret the symptoms of minor illnesses as sinister – such concerns while often unfounded nevertheless need an understanding response from health professionals. As Carol pointed out under such circumstances the GP may be bypassed in favour of what may be perceived as 'a more sympathetic' hearing:

> Yes, and again you know we get women now ringing up years after their treatment ... no matter how far away the treatment is, they do interpret it all back to their cancer experience. And you know they're not hypochondriacs, and GPs should be more aware of the health concerns ... sometimes they do bypass the GP surgery because of that very attitude.
>
> (Carol: Macmillan nurse)

So what kind of follow-up or support service would be valued? This is one of the questions addressed in the following chapters through an attempt to understand how long-term follow-up clinics are experienced and what happens after clinical follow-up terminates – is the cessation a relief that signifies the 'all clear' or does it leave the survivor feeling insecure and without support? There is also the question of why some survivors react in a much more positive way than others. Is this primarily related to their disease type, treatment regime and physical legacy – or does the quality of the experience and preparation for survivorship shape the outcome, and what is the role of family and the informal support network?

The evidence thus far seems to suggest that there are a number of late and long-term effects that survivors of adolescent cancer have to face, some of them – particularly the more clinically related – are better understood, but the psychosocial and emotional ones can only be guessed at on the basis of anecdotal evidence. Even those effects that are well understood, still leave professionals with doubts about how they can best be presented to the young people at the time of diagnosis and treatment. For example: how much should be divulged, when should it be discussed, what support is needed both at the time and in the longer-term, does long-term, ongoing support prevent the survivor from moving on and shape their identity in a negative way? If the appropriate support and preparation for survivorship is given during treatment, might this lessen the need for it in the longer-term?

It is one of the aims of my research to answer these questions and to identify what shapes survivorship in order that the findings may assist in the provision of support and care to maximise a good outcome. However, Levitt and Eshelman (2008) claim that late effects studies have suffered from methodological pitfalls. The more quantitative studies have been affected by differing control groups, selection bias and measurement variances, while they suggest that the quality of life research suffers from inconsistencies in addition to these problems. I hope that I have avoided the pitfalls through the use of in-depth interviews with participants recruited through a variety of approaches, research sites and sampling techniques (see methods appendix) I have built up a substantial database of detailed accounts from a wide range of survivors whose age ranges, illness histories and treatment regimes allow us to take not only an in-depth approach but also a longer view of the changing nature of survivorship amongst a disparate group, many of whom only have their cancer experience in common.

The empirical chapters rely heavily on extensive quotations from the interviews, each participant's name – real or chosen – is in brackets at the end of their quote, and in addition the number of years that have elapsed since their diagnosis is included. If we are to understand whether and how survivorship changes and develops over an extended period it may be helpful to have such a detail readily available. For further details, a summary of participants is included at the beginning of this volume.

So we can see through the concerns of the health professionals in my own research and from the accounts offered through the special edition of *Contact* that survivorship carries with it a variety of challenges. Academic and medical literature, largely from the USA, charts many late and long-term effects; however, the studies on which they are based tend to be quantitative and biomedical rather than qualitative and psychosocial. Nevertheless, their findings are relevant to this volume as, while expressed in different terms, they chart many of the difficulties encountered by the young adult survivors and it is to them that we now turn.

Late and long-term effects studies

To the person seeking information on the survivorship of adolescent cancers, a trawl of the Internet through the input of key words may look promising. For example, the paper 'Posttraumatic Growth in Adolescent Survivors of Cancer and their Mothers and Fathers' (Barakat *et al.* 2006) might be found if the words 'adolescent', 'cancer' and 'survivor' were entered, yet when reading the paper we see that the mean age at diagnosis was 7.9 years, and the survivors are indeed adolescents but what they have survived is a childhood cancer. This is significant as, according to Levitt and Eshelman, information on treatment toxicities is increasingly reported but from adolescent survivors of *childhood* cancer whose results cannot be extrapolated to survivors of adolescent and young adult cancers (2008: 167).

There appears to be a wealth of studies of long-term survivorship that is based primarily on cancers diagnosed and treated in childhood including, for example: Eiser 1998, Hill *et al.* 1998, Kingma *et al.* 2000, Lahteenmaki 2001, Ozono *et al.* 2007, Phipps *et al.* 2000, Prouty *et al.* 2006, Reimers *et al.* 2003, Robison 2005, Steinberg *et al.* 1998, Tyc *et al.* 2001, Van Dongen-Melman 2000 and Wallace *et al.* 2001. This 'gap' in research is commented on by Soliman and Agresta (2008) who report a focus on children or older adults in the survivorship literature. These authors suggest that insufficient data are available to characterise accurately the needs of survivors of adolescent and young adult cancer for whom outcomes are inferior and who they claim are not well served by existing services.

However, while few studies focus specifically on those diagnosed and treated during adolescence and young adulthood there may be 'hidden' evidence about the age group combined with the childhood data. One of the most comprehensive texts on survivorship (Keene *et al.* 2000) is USA-based and focuses on childhood cancer diagnosis. While it does include some cases of adolescent cancers it conflates those diagnosed at an earlier age and life stage using a definition of 'under age 20' (Keene *et al.*: 1) as encompassing 'childhood cancer'. Other studies on survivorship such as that of Little *et al.* (2000) do not specify an age group and discuss the liminality of survivors without specifying age or life stage.

Drew's (2007) mixed method study of illness legacy generated responses from 55 questionnaires and 32 in-depth interviews. While the title of the paper indicates that the participants were the survivors of 'childhood' cancers, upon closer inspection it is clear that a number were diagnosed during their teenage years. However, given that the table provided conflates the age group 11–15 it's not possible to specify exactly how many were teenagers. Nevertheless, most of the quotes from the data used to illustrate the effects are taken from those diagnosed as teenagers. One interesting observation from this study is that those participants with cancers diagnosed as young as 2 years old predictably say: 'being young I couldn't understand what they were saying' (Drew 2007: 288). Yet the recollection, reaction and response of those diagnosed when the implications are much clearer in adolescence and young adulthood, are likely to be significantly different in their ongoing psychological impact.

Mertens *et al.* (2001) suggest that treatment-related complications remain a possibility for up to 25 years after the initial cancer diagnosis, although these figures are based on a study that included both children and adolescent survivors so it is difficult to ascertain if adolescents are at the same risk as young children. Mertens *et al.* (2001) found a 10.8 increase in overall mortality with a statistically significant higher rate of 18.2 in females. The leading cause of death amongst 5 year survivors was a recurrence of the original cancer which accounted for 67 per cent of the deaths. However, subsequent malignancies, cardiac, pulmonary and other causes also contributed. Treatment-related associations were present for subsequent cancer, cardiac and other mortalities. Similarly, Birch *et al.* (2008) suggest that the risk of developing treatment-related second malignancies and organ dysfunction are critical considerations for this age group.

In a press release issued by The Children's Hospital of Philadelphia, a young woman called Barb Lee, who was diagnosed with Ewing's sarcoma at the age of 16 and treated successfully, is reported to have been astonished that years after her initial cancer she was diagnosed with breast cancer an apparently not uncommon side effect in adolescent women who received radiation therapy years before. Barb reported how this experience caused flashbacks to the original treatment and said 'In my wildest dreams I never thought I would face a different cancer one day' (2006). As this press release says the conquest of the disease can be interpreted as a 'mixed victory' because of the way in which both chemotherapy and radiation affect the growing body and mind. Not only were high rates of breast cancer observed in survivors, neurocognitive functioning was also reported to be affected. PTS similar to that seen in war veterans was found in survivors who had both flashbacks and intense anxiety with any minor ache or pain. However, despite increased concern over their health, the same report claims that the PTS can lead to the avoidance of health care such as follow-up visits, mammograms and, paradoxically, other opportunities to reduce the late effects. This raises the questions of: if, when and how an adolescent and young adult cancer patient should be prepared for what may follow later in life.

Silveri *et al.* establish that adolescence has been widely accepted as 'a time for notable alterations in brain functioning' (2004: 363). If such changes are undergone in 'normal circumstances' the experience of having been diagnosed and treated for cancer with all its attendant trauma, stress and challenges to the life trajectory (Grinyer 2007) is likely to compound the effect. In addition the treatment regimes themselves may affect cognitive and brain function in an ongoing way. Cox *et al.* (2005) argue that the late effects of radiation and chemotherapy increase the risk of chronic health problems, yet not only do survivors fail to engage in health-promoting behaviours, they frequently practice high-risk behaviours.

Hollen, Hobbie and Finley examine cognitive late effects factors that relate to decision-making behaviour in adolescents with a history of cancer therapy which is known to have the potential to threaten cognitive function such as intrathecal or high-dose systemic methotrexate. The outcome suggested it could be a predictor of poorer quality decision making which could lead to risk-taking behaviours (1997: 305). Hollen and Hobbie (1993) claim that adolescent survivors may be at greater risk than those in the general population because of the late effects of organ compromise and oncogenesis.

A paper by Hollen, Hobbie, Finley and Hiebert (2001) argues that resiliency is a key factor in risk-taking behaviours and that non-resilient teen survivors were more likely to engage in risk-taking behaviours relating to substance usage. However, such a response may be an understandable reaction to the loss of control experienced through the illness rather than a result of any cognitive impairment or faulty judgement.

Hollen, Hobbie and Finley suggest that risk-taking behaviour information based on potential late effects needs to be offered during follow-up visits and that 'booster programmes' should be available to 'refine decision making skills' (1999: 1475) as a means of reducing risk-taking behaviours. In addition to the cognitive impact on risk behaviours are the effects of the treatments on academic functioning. Phipps *et al.* (2000) study was on children of a significantly younger age at diagnosis and treatment with bone marrow transplant (BMT). Their conclusions are that patients over 6 years of age given a BMT are at minimal risk of late neurocognitive effects. However, addressing the late effects of a different treatment, cranial radiation for acute lymphoblastic leukaemia (ALL), Kingma *et al.* (2000) find it to be clearly associated with a subsequently poorer academic career. Nevertheless, this study too was based on patients treated at a younger age than adolescence.

Zeltzer (1993) lists long-term effects that include: increased health concerns, worries about the development of a secondary cancer, increased somatic complaints and academic problems. Zeltzer's summary of a range of literature suggests that long-term survivors are less likely to be married than siblings, female survivors are more likely to divorce, they are more likely to have left home at a later age than siblings, have a higher chance of experiencing depression, alcoholism or attempting suicide, are more likely to exhibit agitation, restlessness and hyperactivity and to be less successful in their academic pursuits. Fertility concerns were also reported as was an anxiety from the women that their offspring might be adversely affected by their cancer history. The lowest well-being scores were related to those who had been treated with both intrathecal methotrexate and cranial irradiation.

However, to put these negative consequences into context Zeltzer reports that the majority of survivors were well adjusted and leading 'essentially normal lives'. Some positive effects were also reported such as feelings of an increased value in living, increased involvement in social relationships and a coping model that used problem-solving techniques.

Neville (2007) suggests that the long-term consequences can range from the obvious to the subtle but the least obvious are the psychosocial sequelae of surviving teenage cancer. Neville claims that while many studies have been undertaken on late effects the data are 'complex, contradictory and often fraught with the unique psychometric issues of measuring children and adolescents who are distinctly different from adults' (2007: 4). She identifies uncertainty as the greatest psychosocial stressor to families and a significant concern to adolescents. Using Mishel's theory of uncertainty in illness, Neville claims that when uncertainty is interpreted as 'danger', coping strategies are employed that lead to adaptation if effective, but if they are ineffective, maladaptation can lead to psychological distress. However, uncertainty can also, according to Neville, be associated with an appreciation of the fragility and impermanence of life; and in qualitative research young adult survivors of teenage cancers described themselves as 'possessing a maturity beyond their years' (2007: 4). Indeed Spinetta asks if having cancer while a teenager might be helpful rather than harmful in becoming an adult (cited in Neville 2007).

Neville suggests that adaptive denial may be a feature of adolescent response to cancer survival and that this may manifest in a different reaction than with adults, and claims that more research is needed to understand individual progression in later developmental tasks. The need to 'catch up' may be felt, this may be accompanied by a focused career path but difficulties can be experienced in socialisation even years after treatment.

Drew (2007) describes 'an epidemic of survival' with effects that may become apparent as long as 20 or 30 years after treatment. Of the teenage participants in her study of survivors of childhood cancer, she quotes those who speak of the cancer becoming part of their identity, they also experience depression, a sense of loss and the expectation that they should feel 'lucky' to have survived. The physical consequence of weight gain that could lead to eating disorders, hair loss or the loss of sporting prowess and fitness, could all be dispiriting. Uncertainty about fertility and the difficulty in relating to medical professionals was reported and one young woman, diagnosed at 17 suggests that her oncologist did not know how to talk to 'older people', presumably because he was a paediatrician and therefore familiar only with treating children. Drew's participants who had been diagnosed as teenagers also express concern about the lack of preparation about what effects to expect in later life and feel they would have been prepared if they had been given more information.

In an article that is based predominantly on the cancer experience, Miedema *et al.* (2007) identify 'normalcy' as being a goal for survivors of cancer in young adulthood. However, the 'normal' was not necessarily that of their pre-cancer lives. The belief in their 'invincibility' had gone and a 29 year female participant is quoted as follows:

> The thought of trying, how would I ever go back to 'normal' when this is such a life changing event. It was huge and I knew I wasn't the same person from even the mention of it, let alone afterwards.
>
> (Miedema *et al.* 2007: 48)

While all these studies strongly suggest that there are significant late and long-term effects that can result in cognitive, psychological and physical consequences, they are predominantly based on statistical research undertaken by clinicians in a medical setting that do not allow us an in-depth insight into the lived experience of being a survivor of adolescent cancer. Neither do they answer the question of why some survivors adapt better than others in the long term – is this related to their specific illness, their treatment, the setting of care, their age at diagnosis, their gender, or some other imponderable? My research seeks, through in-depth qualitative methods, to understand the phenomenon at a different level so that some of the questions at the start of this chapter can be answered through entering into the life world of the young person. Birch *et al.* (2008) claim survival rates for those between 13 and 24 are improving and have climbed by approximately 11 per cent over the last two decades, thus the need to be able to provide appropriate long-term support becomes increasingly important for the growing number of survivors, about whose needs we currently know little. Soliman and Agresta say the following about the need for research:

> Survivorship studies focusing on the AYA (Adolescents and Young Adults) age group are needed to answer questions about their medical and psychosocial needs. Addressing these issues is essential to achieving the same progress in the AYA cancer population as has been made in other patient populations.
>
> (2008: 61)

This volume aims to contribute to the knowledge that Soliman and Agresta identify as currently being sparse. The following chapters are based on empirical data that address many of the issues raised thus far and include additional themes that arose from the interviews. The next chapter is based on two selected case studies that between them cover a range of issues, but from the contrasting perspectives of a young woman at the start of survivorship, and an older man nearly 50 years after diagnosis. The subsequent chapters are themed and cover issues including: the physical legacy and fear of recurrence; the experience of long-term follow-up clinics and what happens when they are no longer offered; the emotional legacy, how it impacts on the philosophy of life and shapes perspectives; the resistance to victimhood, identity and the positive effects of survivorship; the long-term impact on life plans, careers and finance and finally the effect on fertility.

The study included more than 50 participants thus a wealth of data was collected; but although the interviews are quoted at length, it is only possible to present a fraction of the material gathered, and not all participants can be quoted in each chapter. I have attempted to select quotations that represent the range of experiences and opinions and to indicate where a perspective is typical or atypical. The issues identified are articulated by participants who occupy a range of possible positions along a continuum of responses on that topic; so while the themes and issues raised were addressed by the majority of participants, there is no 'typical participant'. There are many areas of overlap and similarity, but there are also contrasts and contradictions. By following through a participant across the themed chapters it may also be possible to discern internal inconsistencies in one person's narrative. However, that is what long-term survivorship is like; it is not necessarily linear, consistent, wholly positive nor entirely negative.

The participants' only unifying characteristic was that they had been diagnosed with cancer in adolescence/young adulthood, and arguably there is more that divides them in terms of life experience than that which unites them. Nevertheless, the experience of cancer at that age, the identity it confers and the life-long nature of survivorship results in enough consistency across the variety of responses to draw conclusions that contribute to answering the questions posed in this chapter. The implications will be drawn out in the final chapter in order to inform policy, and shape practice, that can provide long-term support to best meet the needs of the survivors of adolescent and young adult cancers.

2   Case studies

When I began the research on long-term survivorship from cancer diagnosed in adolescence or young adulthood, I had no upper age limit in mind but assumed that most participants would be within 10 or 15 years of their treatment having finished. However, I was surprised that recruitment through the charitable sector – where participants were self selected rather than approached by health professionals through follow-up clinics (see methods appendix), long-term survivors of more than 40 years duration volunteered to participate. Clearly the experience of survivorship at 5 years is likely to differ from that at 40 years yet there may also be factors that unite survivors and the quality of survivorship.

In order to understand better the relationship between those at each end of the survivorship spectrum, I have used a purposive sampling technique and selected two case studies. One is a young woman at the start of long-term survivorship and the other is an older man much further along the journey. Of course as Grbich (1999) warns, the researcher's biases need to be clarified; in this instance the selection of the cases occurred late in the data collection period, thus I was able to take an overview of the issues and choose examples that encompassed the majority of the themes addressed in this volume, while also offering a contrasting context. I hope that the presentation and juxtaposition of two such disparate examples illuminates the changing nature of the journey as well as the shared and unchanging aspects of being a survivor of adolescent and young adult cancer.

Why use case studies? The remainder of this volume draws on the interview data collected through the research and, of necessity, fragments the material under themed chapter headings. It is therefore difficult to follow through the entire story of any individual. The organisation of the data in this way has some advantages in that the reader interested in a particular aspect of survivorship can focus on multiple accounts of that theme. However, what this approach lacks is the more holistic nature of the case study where a single person's narrative can be seen in context. As Gilbert (2008) says, the careful selection of a few case studies allows for the examination of detail missing in other methods; and, according to Grbich, this allows for the grounding of a particular phenomenon. Robson argues that a case study is defined solely in terms of a specific case in its context and can be 'as pre-structured or "emergent" as you wish' (1995: 149). In this case it is part of an exploratory exercise to assist an understanding of a range of issues as they might apply to the wider sample. The added comparators of age, gender and length of time since treatment and diagnosis, represent the range of the survivorship continuum. Robson argues that such an approach is helpful in research where there is little previous knowledge to guide the researcher as to what to look for.

I have taken the interview material and edited it, of necessity, as both the interviews were lengthy, but I have allowed the participants' voices to be heard in the first person rather than summarise their stories myself. Ruth's mother, Anne, was present at Ruth's interview and I have included some interjections from her as I feel it is significant that where she prompted Ruth be made explicit because it allows some insight into the dynamics between a young adult survivor and her mother. The result is that these accounts offer a glimpse of what survivorship has meant to two people with very different perspectives Ruth, at the age of 20 and Bob at the age of 62.

Ruth's story

Brief biography: Ruth was diagnosed at 14 with anaplastic large cell lymphoma (ALCL); she was 20 when I interviewed her. At the time of the interview she was an undergraduate music student. She had previously withdrawn from the nursing degree begun upon leaving school after having decided that her original choice of reading medicine was no longer an option following her illness.

Ruth

It's been 5 years now. Well I finished [treatment] *in June 2002, I haven't had any treatment since then. It* [follow-up] *was every month, and then every 2 months. And then it went to 3 months, and then 6 months, and then a year ... I don't know whether I should have seen my consultant – he said that I should have seen the long-term side effects doctor. He's someone else. And that's every year. So I'm seeing her this week. So it was a bit confusing.*

I try not to think about it [follow-up]. *I don't really want to go back anymore. I don't think I used to mind, but when it got to about a year I hadn't been back for such a long time, I think then it seems different. It's just like ... Oh I don't know ... it's part of the past now. I don't really want to go back. And when you're back it's like you've never been away really. But I don't really like going back. I'm glad when it's over and I'm sort of back in reality ... it's like you go in and you sit down with all the little kids. It's quite funny really because it's as if you should be the parent ... it's a bit weird. Especially when I did nurse training ... I could be a student nurse really … we do normally end up waiting, but we always have … they're quite busy.*

I think I thought that it (having cancer) *must have happened for a reason, so I should do nursing. And … it's all linked in with the control thing, and like sort of making my life perfect again. And just … yes, and I sort of thought through logically what I could do, and what I wanted to do. And I didn't … I think with the flute playing I thought well I won't be able to get a job at the end of it, so I may as well do nursing … and it went from being a doctor … and then I thought well I can't do medicine it's just too difficult. But that took a long time for me to realise as well … and then it went onto nursing and … I mean I remember the first time I went into hospital and I was just really scared, I didn't want to go in. So it changed a lot within that year. And I don't know in a way if it was me, in a really weird way, trying to hold on to the experience and thinking how can life go on normally? Like how can I just forget all that and just pretend that it didn't happen. So I may as well go and do nursing. But I just used to say to myself no, no it's the right thing to do because I'm going to help other people and I have … and it is true in a way, and maybe one day I might go back to it.*

I've had cognitive difficulties. So like reading and … well particularly the reading … I can read out loud and it sounds like I'm reading fine. And anyone listening will say oh yes there's nothing wrong. But for me to actually be absorbing what it's saying, the information, it's quite difficult. And I had to find myself – this was when I was at uni last year – and I found myself reading over and over the same sentence like three times or something, and visualising each word … at first I just thought it was me not concentrating, but then after a while I spoke to mum about it and got an educational assessment, and it turned out that there were quite a few … structural things … like writing an essay … it's quite funny really, I'll get all the different bits of information, put them all down on a piece of paper, and then I won't be able to write the actual essay … just put it all together really. And then I'll also struggle with just general attention span I think. And when I'm talking, I'll be talking to someone and I'll forget what I'm saying … my mind will totally go off it. It's quite funny sometimes, but when you're in a conversation and you need to be focused, it's quite difficult … Well I think it's from the methotrexate, because it was intrathecal. And they say that it can cause that (cognitive problems) *… I think that if we'd have known … I know they sort of say they shouldn't tell you it's a possibility because you'll start to imagine it. But I don't know if … I think if you would they'd tell you, but if it was a real problem like that it's better to know before than to sort of struggle along with it.*

I think that does affect you socially … I think one of the main things is just the fact that no-one really knows what you've been through. And yes … that's the main thing … that I always felt that I had to tell people that it was like a sort of … some … like it sort of made my past, which is true, but I don't think it is necessary anymore. I used to feel, straight away, as soon as I met someone, it was something I had to get done, and tell them all. But now I think you'll tell them in your own time … but I'm not sure. I think there is a danger … because I went out with someone actually and … I think he 'googled' my name and found all those articles on the Internet. And he said to me that he didn't want to read them because I think he was scared that he would victimise me and feel sorry for me. And that would affect how he viewed me. And at the time I was thinking, 'What, what is he going on [about] … Just read the stupid thing.' But now I understand what he was talking about … It did annoy me sometimes, like when … because there's some horrible pictures of me as well. And that really got to me sometimes, I was just because it's hard to … although it seems quite real, it's like you know what happened in your head as well, and you always think oh it was worse than that, it was worse than what I wrote. And you think that people get the wrong ideas as well. And it's difficult, but yes, I think I'd rather have it on there anonymously … I'd rather tell them to read it instead of them find it, I don't know.

When you go to the GP, I think they're over cautious. And they sort of worry straight away I think – depending on who you get – and send you straight back to the hospital. A few weeks ago, I didn't to be honest think it was [a relapse] because I know what my consultant said it's a really slim chance of relapsing at this stage. And I'm sure that I would know if there was something really wrong.

But it was the fact that I went there and then the GP said, you know it was because I had glands under my arms … and that's what I had at the beginning … I thought they weren't glands, they felt more like from shaving or something like that. And yes, so I went to see the GP and he said, 'No, no, they are glands' and sort of … he wasn't that worried because he said they're only small, but ended up sending me back to the hospital to be on the safe side anyway.

Ruth's mother Anne

But you were actually worried Ruth weren't you, underneath it? Because … there've been other times when she's had swollen glands and in the past – especially early on – I would panic straight away. I panic far less now though; I'm much more laid back about it now, but vigilant. But this time Ruth persisted …

Ruth

I didn't feel like it was [a relapse] underneath, but then I think it's because the GP … because you think well they must know better than you. And when they seem so sure that is like glands and not something else ...

When I was actually ill I didn't really think that much about the future, about ... it was just like surviving really. And then after I was ill, it sort of went a bit obsessive and controlled ... and I just concentrated because I'd put on a lot of weight from steroids and stuff. And I think I concentrated on losing weight, and got really obsessive. I didn't really think about it [weight] *before I was ill. But then when I was and I had steroids and I put weight on, I was just like, no I've got to lose weight now. And that's when it became a bit too controlled.*

And I think that's my personality, I'm a bit of a perfectionist, and it's really bad because it just ... it did get out of hand. And so that took over for a while ... that was all through sixth form it sort of took over my life. And then I went to uni and it was still there, but it [being at uni] *sort of helped to deal with that. And yes, I can honestly say that only really finished ... that whole obsessiveness ... at the end of that first year at uni. But now, yes I think I've just ... I am quite controlled in sort of everything that I do.*

I'm definitely not scared of death now, because that's what I thought when I had that scare the other week. It's more like getting things right in life I think that I worry about now, because ... I don't know, maybe it's because I just ... I'm more aware of the fact that I only have one chance ... and like with the fact that things went wrong, and decisions that I've made that have gone wrong, I think that's why I sort of have to reassure myself all the time that I'm doing the right thing. So I don't know ... I don't know whether ... whether it's a positive thing or a negative thing ... I don't know.

I've got Raynaud's disease which is cold hands and cold extremities and stuff. And general cold, but sometimes I think that that's partly as well due to the fact that I lost too much weight ... and then when I went to clinic ... at first they said 'oh no it's not due to the chemo that you had', and ... then they sort of say 'oh no it is'. And it's quite confusing sometimes what is and what isn't ... not that it actually matters now. We were talking to my consultant and I mentioned it again, and he actually typed it in [vinblastine and Raynaud's disease], *and said, 'oh yes, you're right' ... You sometimes think that you're making a bit ... of a fuss really and you shouldn't mention it.*

I think my decision-making process has definitely been affected by ... because in fact that's probably the main thing, from just missing out a year. It's not the fact that you've been through a sort of death, but more that I think, as well, you miss out on just normal growing up experiences, and just normal socialising and what normal teenagers would go through. I think you think, well they're not really important because you know you've been through a lot worse. But yes, I think it does matter in the end. It means you have to catch up, and you don't have the space to catch up.

It's like in the one sense you know a lot about the end of life, like an old woman would know, but in other ways you're not used to normal life, and just living every day. Yes, I think that's probably one of the things that have come out.

I think it [a self help group or support group for long-term survivors] *would be quite good actually because ... just because for the people that have been through the same thing as you ... because one of the big things is feeling different to all your friends. I think it affected my mum a lot, the fact that they changed my doctor ... the fact that we were going to some-one different.*

Anne

Well it's not so much that Ruth, I think it was the fact that it was ... it wasn't made clear what was happening. And this five year check-up, I think for me, was a big thing. It was the end of the protocol, and it's as if we've been holding our breath ever since you were first diagnosed. I couldn't understand ... I really did react didn't I when we went that day Ruth. And I found myself on the verge of tears, and I couldn't understand why I was reacting so strongly. But I realise that from the time Ruth was diagnosed and we were given this awful news ... we were told, don't get ahead of yourselves, there's no guarantees. And then when she was in remission, we were told again, you can't ... you know there's still a strong chance of recurrence. And that was the message that we were given con-stantly. Not just while she was on treatment but afterwards, and going back for scans, knowing what they were checking for ... it was as if we'd never been told well you can begin to breathe more easily ... it was the end of the protocol and suddenly there was nothing ... just a cancelled appointment!

Ruth

But now it's just like ... it sort of seems to be over and that's what they seem to focus on. And I don't think they really ... think of the psycho-logical effects ... I think that I felt more, that I've thought about it too much in a way, [the consultant] *said something about me thinking more than any other person, and I sort of felt, oh I think too much. And I thought well maybe ... maybe I do just think too much about it, and like yes I have survived and ... I don't know really.*

Anne

But recently he [the consultant] *said that he was quite grateful for all that we'd shared, because he said that it's given him an insight into the long-term effects. But I think, especially as follow-up visits get less and less, and obviously the main thing is checking for any recurrence and any very serious late effects, that there isn't time, in that short space, to really explore what are the psychological effects – how are you coping. So I don't think it's really that they aren't concerned, I think it's just that within the structure of … the service provided, they can only do so much.*

Ruth

I think that [my fertility is] alright because they said that otherwise my periods wouldn't have come back. And, I don't know … I mean they said there's always a chance, but that's what they say about everything that there's always a chance … they said there's a chance of early menopause in like late twenties, but I don't really think about that.

Anne

Ruth, you haven't said anything about the symptoms of Post Traumatic Stress (PTS), you know when you were [nursing]. When you were passing the children's oncology ward, and how you felt when you went on the placement … and how you felt. You talked about long-term survivors … there was a conference actually in Scotland in December, for long-term survivors, and Ruth was going to go on that. And you didn't go because you felt that it would be too upsetting at the time. You were … you said you would have just cried the whole time, and you didn't know anybody else.

Ruth

I think so, like I think that … I don't know if there's anything say on TV or just generally, if you think back to it, it's just quite upsetting really. And I mean I don't … I don't know if there is a right way to deal with it or if there is anyway to deal with it really … I think probably the hardest thing is that when you remember these things and it's just like … and people don't understand, and you can't really explain it either because it's like you've been there, but the only people who do understand are the people who have been there or who were with you at the time. So I think it is quite hard to sort of explain in words, and I … so it gets quite frustrating if you think that people aren't understanding you. And they're just like saying, 'Oh no, no you've survived though haven't you, you've survived.' And that's quite difficult.

Bob's story

Brief biography: Bob was diagnosed at 14 with non-Hodgkin's lymphoma; he was 62 when I interviewed him. Bob is a GP, married with grown up children. At the time of the interview he had taken early retirement from his General Practice after an amputation, but had returned to work part time.

Bob

I was 14, nearly 15, when the cancer was diagnosed ... I started developing pain in my right leg. I was a very active hill walker at the time, and I found that walking was becoming quite difficult. This all happened [in] November 1960. There were no suitable treatment facilities in Aberdeen, so I was referred to Edinburgh, and spent six weeks as a patient in Edinburgh having radiotherapy ... It was a non-Hodgkin's lymphoma ... in the lower end of the femur ... I've been very lucky, surviving.

It's [the illness experience] made a huge difference. I think firstly it reinforced my previous desire to become a doctor ... because [of] the episodes in hospital, I realised that some of the care was good, some was not very good. And I felt there was areas where I'd like to try and see if I couldn't do better than what I'd experienced. And so I did medicine, and because I'd been through a cancer illness, right through my medical school I had a special interest in cancer, and actually was a joint author and patient on a couple of papers on cancer before I graduated. And then as I post grad I did cancer research, and continued to be involved in that. So from that point of view it has strongly influenced it.

I've picked up experiences when I was having my first treatment of little things where the people were saying things to you didn't realise how offensive they were. I'd been in this orthopaedic ward for four weeks. And as I was leaving the ward to go to the ambulance the ward sister took my crutches away from me, which were my only way of mobility. And she says, 'You can't take these with you.' I said, 'But I'm not allowed to walk.' She said, 'Oh we've had this before, if crutches leave this ward we never see them again.' And so I was stranded. And there I was trying to get to Edinburgh. And she handed me a urinal to use on the train, because I wouldn't be able to get to the toilet on the train. Now a 14-year-old guy doesn't enjoy that very much.

When I got to Edinburgh, because I didn't have crutches, I was wheeled into the ward lying – and I was physically well, I was well in myself – lying on a trolley facing up. And this ward sister looked down on me and says, 'You should have been here last week, and you've missed the professor's ward round' – as if it was my fault, you know. And I remember these were the words of welcome.

So the way that you leave your patients, and the way you greet them, has become far more important to me, because the wrong word said can make such a difference ... And so I hope I consciously try to make people feel at ease, and I give them an opportunity to have a dialogue about anything that may be concerning them. And certainly because of my very frequent periods in hospitals and outpatients, I've seen so many things that offended me, and knowing these other patients have been treated, etc., that I think I'm a wee bit more conscious about being on the receiving end, and what that means. And I hope I've modified how I cope with it.

I think the down side is I have such a focus on cancer, it may well be that I've neglected other areas of post graduate training, because they're not quite so much of an interest to me. I'm very just focused on one thing, so perhaps poor folk that come in with a sore ear don't get quite the same level of expertise as they would do if they had a potential cancer you know.

I had the embarrassing situation of never having been told my diagnosis. My parents were. My mother was keen that I shouldn't be told, because that was the way things were in the early 1960s ... as I went through medical school and it was only when I was going to Hammersmith, one of the oncology professors there said I think we should look at the slides again. So we had the slides reviewed it was a non-Hodgkin's lymphoma ... that would have been probably 1991/92, that I had final confirmation of what the diagnosis was. Over 30 years later, yes.

I think [long-term follow-up] is highly random ... does follow-up mean that you'll get better survival, in terms of length of survival? We don't have good information on that for most cancers. And so follow-up programmes are often just things scribbled out on the back of an envelope ... but do we get it right, and who should be doing it, is still very much an open debate ... I think the positive thing has been that in the last few years cancer has now moved to being seen as, like surviving diabetes and things like that, as a chronic disease entity. And then we can take examples of how we manage other chronic diseases – and some of them are now being done quite well. And diabetes is an example of that, where there is a definite system set-up whereby there can be long-term surveillance, which is appropriate for the needs of the individual – because people don't want to be going to clinics all the time, and they do want the condition to be reviewed ... you have to continue doing research into what makes the difference in terms of survivorship, and for breast cancer you say an annual mammogram does that. But there's what may make a difference to the well-being of the person ... have an open door policy ... when they feel either there's something going wrong or they feel they need support, have a specialist nurse, or a number they always can carry with them to phone, where there is an open door to go in.

And I'm a good example of [Post Traumatic Stress (PTS)] because my treatment was in the Western Infirmary ... Western General in Edinburgh, and I go round all the cancer centres as part of my Scottish Cancer Group post, and I still have a very, very uneasy feeling going into that building ... I was doing an official visit there not more than three months ago, and going along the corridor of the ward where I was in, and looking into the room where I was, it puts a shiver down your spine ... So if I'm feeling that with the sort of ease that I wander through hospitals, then other people who are far less au fait with hospitals must feel it far more ... I think that, you know, follow-up's a real problem.

I have maintained an interest in cancer services. I was the first lead cancer GP in a lead cancer team in the UK, sponsored by Macmillan, and I now chair the Scottish Cancer Group. So I've been heavily involved with cancer service development. From my own career point of view, I think – I hope – that my many hospital experiences over the years have modified my approach to patients.

I went through medical school and thoroughly enjoyed it, and carried on to ... went to Glasgow to do some cancer research, met Joan who is my wife, and we got married very quickly. And eventually went into general practice, and about ... so that was 1973, and in about 1975 suddenly my leg started to swell. And I was very anxious at that stage that it was a recurrence of tumour, because I had no follow-up from my cancer treatment.

I re-established contact with the local cancer service, and was taken in for a lymph angiogram, and it showed that in fact the swelling was due to the radiotherapy – blocking the lymphatics of the right leg. And you can actually see a straight line where the field of radiotherapy was, and the blockage ... So that was a chronic problem.

I remember one night in 1988 I was on call ... I went to bed on a Sunday night, absolutely well. I had the usual very full weekend of work, and went to bed at about midnight. And half an hour later woke up shivering. And what had happened was that I'd developed septicaemia from an infection bedding into the bone at the tumour site – what had been the tumour site. And of course with the leg being swollen cellulitis developed in the leg, in the soft tissue. So it wasn't just the bone, but it was the soft tissues. And from 1988 onwards I have had recurrent episodes of very severe infection, resulting in long periods off work, and while straight forward antibiotic therapy wasn't eradicating the problem, I was persuaded to consider a surgical approach to this.

So I had two three-stage operations in Dundee, and neither of them succeeded. Then I went to London to see an eminent professor there. He felt he could do the same operation in a different way, so I was up and down to London, going through that. And again that failed to succeed, so eventually my consultants here in Fife said I think you should stay on antibiotics permanently, and we'll see how we go. And so in all I was on antibiotics for 14 years.

Then almost exactly seven years ago from now I fell while I was out with my dog. A very gentle fall, but my leg fell apart. The leg broke, and this is a pathological fracture through the tumour site. And the fracture inevitably failed to heal. Well the local orthopaedic service took some persuading that that was going to be what happened. And I got frustrated with the service here, and e-mailed the National Orthopaedic Hospital, and made contact with a brilliant chap down there, who agreed to take me on and investigate me. And he eventually took my femur out and put a metal one in its place. And we really thought we'd cracked it – walking well, feeling great. But when the antibiotics stopped the infection came back again.

So that takes us through to the early 2002 metalwork – this huge bit of metalwork got infected. I was looking pretty rotten. So I tried to get back to work but failed, and had to take early retirement from practice. And that finally took place in July of 2002. And in the October of 2002 yet again, once through the night, despite being on antibiotics, I became very ill and got myself back to hospital in Dundee, where there was a good infectious diseases unit. And they poured antibiotics into me for ten days. But by then I was still looking absolutely awful, and decided the only way forward was for them to amputate. So I asked them to do that, and they readily agreed. And so that took place, I think it was 1st November, 2002. And since then my health's been fantastic. I'm so much better.

I've lost my leg now, in the last six years. And so in some ways that's been negative, but in fact if you actually analyse what's happened in my life since amputation, then maybe I've done even more since than I did before. So all these things are on one level are bit negative, in other ways they've been very positive.

Clearly now looking back, there was several key points where I should have said okay game's up, let's just go for it. But I was at a stage in my career where retirement would have been financially really embarrassing. And it would have had a dire effect as a family. And of course my family as they've grown up, never knowing whether I'm going to be there on a morning or not, because often I was whipped off to hospital through the night. And you know, this is their ... one of their recollections of their growing up, was where's dad going to be tomorrow, you know.

[There's been a] *huge, huge absolutely huge emotional impact – great uncertainty over us all ... and for long periods in hospital in London when the family were up here, and the cost of that and the emotional separation and all the rest – quite a major thing ... we are a close family. I think in some ways we've become closer ... we have our ups and downs like every other family. But we've tried very hard to involve the family in all the decisions that we've been making, and make them understand what's been going on. And you know, in 1988 my youngest daughter was only seven. So it's quite a lot for a seven-year-old to take on board – the dad who seems unburstable is suddenly in hospital and looking very poorly. And that's it. So I think it's just by explaining and giving time, and you know involving them fully in the whole thing. And it's for others to judge whether we've done it well or not.*

I've now come back into medicine with my amputation, because I had an insurance policy ... a year after the amputation, when I was struggling to cope with the prosthetic – which I still struggle to cope with, I barely ever use it ... they sent a nurse to the house who spent an hour with me, and she said we think you may be fit to return to work. And by that stage of course I'd resigned from my practice; I'd no obvious place to go to. And it was all a bit of a shock. And I was still going through further investigations, because of the circulation problems in my stump at that stage. And it was just at the wrong time.

But anyway I reflected on it, and thought well I always loved my work, and maybe this is a good idea. I never wanted to retire at that age, it had been forced upon me. So anyway I went to the local post graduate Dean for General Practice and presented him with the problem. He agreed to fund me to go back to a practice of his choosing for six months, as an extra pair of hands, funded by himself, and by his department. And so I was put to practice seven miles away from here, and it turned out to be a dream practice, fantastic. And I'm now a part-time salaried GP working with a really great team of doctors.

So ... that's been very positive too, and I just love my three sessions a week back in practice. And it's given me the ability to get involved in the Scottish Cancer Group, and I'm involved with the Clinical Studies Development Group with the NCRI, where the Teenage Cancer Trust is obviously heavily involved, and involved with lots of other wee bits and pieces up here, all cancer related. And done a lot of charity work as well.

Well there's clearly been times when I've not been able to [go walking] ... but we do probably more walking now than we ever did. I've got the best crutches you can get, and I can walk up hills and down dales, and in the last ... well since my amputation we've twice done what's called the Fife Coastal Walk, from Dundee to Edinburgh, which is 108 miles. Once to raise money for Macmillan, and once for the Maggie's Charity. And we had great fun doing that. So we do ... try and do a couple of walks, decent walks, every weekend and get outside as much as possible. And so walking is still very important.

I suppose financially had I stayed in practice I'd have been able to benefit more from the massive increase in GP's salaries that have taken place over the last few years. But as against that I'm comfortably off with the ... you know I get my superannuation, my insurance money, and what I get from the practice, I'm comfortably off. And I think my quality of life is really very good. And so yes, there's not that many negative things about it.

I think because I was 14 when it happened, and before I was applying for major bits of funding, I was more than a ten year survivor, some of the insurance companies were quite happy to take me on. They reckoned that in a childhood cancer, if you got to ten years the chances were you were cured. And so you know, that was it, I had ... I think my first life insurance that I took on was heavily loaded. And then I went to have a broker who got me quite good life insurance, at normal rate. And my permanent health insurance was really set-up as part of a package with the practice. But other people are definitely struggling, and I think you know, if you have a recent cancer diagnosis you're very much up against it. And you know I've been very fortunate in being in a sector of employment where you get six months sickness – absence without loss of salary. Things like that, so that I'm highly privileged.

I'm probably Chair of the Scottish Cancer Group because I'm a cancer survivor. It was politically correct for them to appoint somebody in my position. And it was helpful to them to have somebody who came in with a fair degree of background knowledge of cancer service development, and also as a doctor. But of these three things, it was the cancer survivorship that was the thing that opened the door to this. You know I've just been asked to join the clinical network for Childhood and Young Persons Cancer in Scotland, a national network. And again they've made it very clear that one of the key items that induced them to invite me was cancer survivorship.

I was in a group looking at long-term survivorship of childhood cancer, and could only participate partly in that because I was in hospital quite a bit of the time the group was working. But again, follow-up was one of the things we really struggled with, because of the lack of evidence, but realising for a lot of childhood cancers, in particular the technical issues of hormones and all the rest, were so intense that some follow-up was [necessary] ... and we made a very strong recommendation there should be for childhood cancer, life-long follow-up, appropriate to the individual.

But of course that ends up with paediatricians looking after people in their forties, unless an alternative regime is set-up. And nobody seems to have come up with any regime where they're doing it in a satisfactory way ... An awful lot could be done within primary care. But the difficulty then is ensuring that each GP that's involved has the skills, the understanding, the background knowledge to handle things appropriately. And that's almost impossible to achieve ... And when you do speak to survivors, well my experience is some of them find it very difficult, because sometimes they've had a bad experience with primary care ... you know in terms of delaying diagnosis in the first place, and therefore they have lost trust.

I've had my period of hypochondriasis without any doubt at all when I've over interpreted symptoms, and pushed for perhaps more investigation than the thing warranted. And I can only justify that on the basis of the fact that you feel very vulnerable at times. And it's the lack of knowledge of what's going on that causes the greatest anxiety ... [but] I've been very fortunate because from all the major systems in my body, apart from my leg, I've remained fairly well despite my recurrent septicaemias and all the rest ... And so at the end of the day I'm fit and well, and probably in better health now than I've been for many years. And so I'm in a fairly unique situation for somebody who has had another type of tumour, you know involving liver, lung, or whatever, they may well be in a state of quite severe debility, and they will be viewing life in a very different way from myself, a person with energy and keen to take on every new challenge. And so I'm not able to speak for them in any way.

I think from the GPs point of view, I think you know, what we've got to offer the patient is continuity of care, and that is under severe threat by everything the professionals are doing with the bigger practices, no out of hours cover and all the rest of it ...

Comparing the cases

What can we learn from the two accounts provided? Ruth and Bob had both been diagnosed with types of lymphoma but these took very different forms with dissimilar symptoms, treatments and physical legacies. They also occupy different positions on the survivorship continuum, and are at different life stages yet their experiences echo one another's in a number of ways.

Firstly it is clear that for both of them the illness and its legacy has become part of their identity. There is perhaps unsurprisingly more willingness for Bob to embrace this identity through his work in the cancer field than for Ruth, earlier in the process, seeking to put it behind her, though Ruth has identified herself in the semi-public domain of the Internet as a survivor and written first hand accounts of her experiences. It may be that the further away from the cancer experience and the more secure other identities become, both personal and professional, the easier it is to incorporate survivorship as central.

Both Ruth and Bob experience something akin to Post Traumatic Stress Disorder (PTSD) under certain circumstances. Despite Bob's familiarity with the medical environment, a visit to the hospital where he was treated more than 40 years earlier can precipitate strong negative emotions. While it appears that Bob was offered no long-term follow-up, his PTSD like reaction to revisiting his place of treatment suggests that it would have caused him some distress had long-term follow-up been offered in that location. Ruth also spoke of her reluctance to go back for more check-ups and said she just wanted to move on. Despite this it seems from her mother's comments that the cessation of the regular health checks would leave them with no support and with feelings of insecurity. It is interesting that while Ruth experiences similar PTSD type triggers, from for example an unexpected TV programme, it was her mother who 'reminded' Ruth that this was the case when she was on her student placement in a hospital. It is also clear that she has avoided predictable triggers such as the survivors conference which instead of promising peer support in prospect made her fear precipitation into distress.

There were ongoing physical legacies from both Ruth and Bob's cancers but these took very different forms. For Bob the persistent pain and discomfort from his leg, accompanied on occasion by septicaemia, had punctuated and permeated his professional and personal life. It had affected to some extent his career choices and had impacted upon his children who had to come to terms with his sudden hospitalisations. Ruth's impairments include Raynaud's syndrome, a condition that affects the circulation and can cause numbness in the fingers, which for a flute player and an aspiring professional musician – as she now is – may have serious implications. But Ruth's physical legacies have been accompanied by cognitive impairment thought to have been precipitated by the drug regime with which she was treated during her illness. It remains to be seen if Ruth's health continues to be affected for as long as Bob's has been, but interestingly, despite the trauma of amputation, it appears that Bob's health is better now than it has been for many years suggesting that improvement may be possible even at a later stage.

It seems that neither Ruth nor Bob had been well prepared for the ongoing physical implications – while in the period of time that has elapsed since Bob's diagnosis and treatment in the 1960s there has been a change in culture to a much more 'open awareness' context, it appears that in Ruth's case her physicians are relying on her to tell them what the impact has been as they remain largely unaware of some of the late effects. Both Ruth and Bob have experienced something akin to hypochondria on occasion and understandably worry about their health and the implications of what others might perceive to be minor ailments. This concern was mirrored by their GPs who, knowing their medical history, took precautions to establish that their seemingly trivial symptoms did not herald a relapse.

During Bob's interview it became apparent that he and his wife had children, and that infertility had not been a problem for him. While Ruth is optimistic that the return of her periods indicates that she too will be fertile, there is the possibility of an early menopause which could mean that, even if she is not in a relationship and while she is still relatively young, she may have to make early choices in order to preserve her options for future procreation. Here the gender difference is relevant as her reproductive life may have been artificially shortened in a way that would not be the same for a male survivor.

Both Bob and Ruth had chosen careers in medicine as a result of their cancers. For Bob, his negative treatment at the hands of insensitive health professionals had informed his clinical practice over a lifetime as a doctor. It was Bob's intention to improve on the care he had been given. For Ruth the motivation appears to have been more akin to a determination to repay the 'debt' of care by undertaking training to be able to give care herself. The outcome for her had not been as positive. Deciding that after her illness her original hope to be a doctor was unfeasible, she opted instead for nursing. However, the combination of stress and trauma she experienced in the hospital environment, coupled with the problems associated with her cognitive impairment, made this choice untenable. Her current role as a music student may in fact have been the better route all along, but it seems that a driving need to 'do the right thing' and her tendency to perfectionism propelled her into a profession that was possibly the least suitable. Certainly it shaped her educational and career choices, as it did Bob's, at a crucial time in their lives.

It is not yet possible to assess the long-term financial impact of Ruth's illness but she had begun a course that it transpired was not right for her, and this in itself has carried a financial implication, even if it's only that she will be entering the labour market later than she might have hoped. There are indications from Bob's account that had he not been in the medical profession financial issues may have been a problem, and even within what he describes as a fortunate and privileged profession, there have still been financial implications.

Both Bob and Ruth articulated the lack of ongoing support that lies outside the clinical follow-up and welcomed the possibility that such a service might be developed for people in their position to dip into as necessary. It also seems clear from both of them that this needs to be situated outside the medical environment as both spoke of the stress caused by returning to their place of care. Despite this expressed need, it was clear that once long-term follow-up had ceased there was an anxiety about being left without any reassurance – indeed this seems to have been something never made available to Bob at any stage.

The emotional impact on both Ruth and Bob is clear. As Bob acknowledges it has been 'huge' and for Ruth this manifested in a tendency towards obsessiveness that contributed to an eating disorder. Yet alongside this Ruth acknowledges that in some ways she became old beyond her years with a maturity that set her apart from her peers. Implicit throughout both accounts are indications that life choices and attitudes had been shaped by the illness. While neither claimed an 'epiphany' or 'moment of truth' there are nevertheless indications of an altered philosophical outlook – as Ruth said 'I'm more aware of the fact that I only have one chance'.

Bob reported more positive outcomes than Ruth, but that may be because he has been able to view the experience from a greater distance and see the shape of his subsequent life and achievements in context. However, Bob did not learn that his illness had been 'cancer' until several years after the event; whether this has shaped his approach to life is unclear. Such a revelation could have damaged his trust in the medical profession, particularly if he had not already embarked on a medical career. Alternatively the effect may have been protective at a vulnerable time of life when he might not have had the maturity to deal with the information. At the very least this raises questions about how maturity and the capacity to deal with the diagnosis of life-threatening illness can be judged during a life stage when age alone is not a predictor of the ability to manage such information.

While the quality of survivorship may change and develop over the years and while the detail may vary according to illness type and the legacies associated with specific treatments, it is clear that survivorship is life-long and that at the transitional life stage of young adulthood the experience of cancer has a distinct and lasting impact. All the issues raised through these two case studies are closely examined throughout the discussion in the following chapters that draw heavily upon the accounts of the research participants and use their own words to illustrate their experiences.

Key points

The case studies addressed

* Post Traumatic Stress (PTS)
* Psychological impact
* Physical legacies
* Impact on life plans and family
* The shaping of life choices
* The emotional impact of returning to the place of care
* Ambivalence over clinical follow-up
* The need for ongoing support

---

3 The physical legacy and the fear of recurrence

According to Soliman and Agresta cancer sub types in this age group vary in comparison with other age groups (2008: 56). Ninety five per cent of cancers in young adults comprise of: Hodgkin's lymphoma, melanoma, testicular cancer, female genital tract malignancies, thyroid cancer, soft tissue sarcomas, non-Hodgkin's lymphoma, leukaemia, brain and spinal cord tumours, breast cancer, bone sarcomas, and non gonadal germ cell tumours. Soliman and Agresta claim that the challenges experienced by patients during treatments for such malignancies persist well after the treatments have ended but point out that much of the data cited reflects the experience of children or older adults, yet there is evidence that late and long-term effects can depend on the age at initial diagnosis.

Langeveld and Arbuckle (2008) document studies that suggest that two-thirds of survivors experience at least one chronic or late occurring complication and one-third have serious or life-threatening complications. According to Levitt and Eshelman (2008) as successful multi-modality treatment is not tumour specific, normal tissue is damaged and it is in the 'after cure' period when the risk of relapse is receding that such damage requires assessment and management.

Soliman and Agresta (2008) chart a number of late effects including second malignancies associated with chemotherapy and radiotherapy, but say that the exact magnitude of the risk is not well understood as there are few studies that focus on the age group. There is also a higher risk of second primary cancers due to the intensity of the initial treatment and the longer life expectancy in the age group, but genetic factors may also play a part. Late cardiac mortality has also been described as a risk of the cardiotoxicity associated with anthracyclines (Soliman and Agresta 2008: 57).

One of the problems with attempting to review the impact of the physical legacy is of course the wide variety of illnesses and tumour types that cancer survivors have experienced. Coupled with this, the difference in treatment regimes and the legacies of chemotherapy, radiotherapy and surgery may result in very different long-term symptoms or late effects. This chapter could have been organised around a list of ongoing and late physical effects – indeed very few of the participants did not tell me of some form of long-term or late

physical effect. However, rather than approach the empirical data by presenting a litany of ongoing physical symptoms, I have instead tried to draw
out the implications and meanings that those effects have on the way in which
they are experienced.[5]

During my previous research I spoke to health professionals who expressed
concern and uncertainty about how the young adult with cancer can be best
prepared for what to expect in later life as result of their cancer and its treatment. This uncertainty is in part due to the age of the young person at the time
of diagnosis and treatment – for example, levels of comprehension and maturity may be difficult to ascertain. In addition there can be concern that should
all the possible sequelae be specified, aggressive treatments might be rejected
as not worth going through if the resulting quality of life could not be assured.
Even though a cure might be possible, the price could be perceived as too
high. This age group – unlike children – would normally have the right to
make their own decisions and would also be aware that the results of those
decisions could be carried with them for decades. Long-term physical consequences and later effects at this age have profound implications for many
aspects of life that are not limited to the physical, they can also have far-
reaching social and emotional dimensions that may be life-long. So, taking
these concerns into consideration, how can young people be best informed
and prepared? This chapter also examines these issues through the interview
data and first hand accounts of survivorship.

Readers may note that there are a disproportionate number of extracts
from survivors of lymphomas in this chapter. This is partly because
Hodgkin's lymphoma is a cancer commonly experienced in young adulthood
and there are many lymphoma survivors' stories in this book; indeed some of
my recruitment was through the Lymphoma Association (see methods
appendix). It is also the case that I happened to tap into a pool of Hodgkin's
lymphoma survivors all of whom were women facing the prospect of breast
cancer resulting from mantle field radiotherapy years earlier (Soliman and
Agresta 2008). The causal link is explained as follows by Zablotska *et al.*:

> Introduction of intensive radiotherapy and chemotherapy to treat
> Hodgkin's disease (HD) three decades ago dramatically changed survival
> times … long-term sequelae of treatment have become increasingly
> important as patients now survive for several decades … several studies
> looked at breast cancer incidence and mortality, the most frequently seen
> second malignancy following treatment for HD … in summary, it
> appears that radiation treatment for HD increases the risk of second
> malignancies … a major increase in risk appears at 10 to 14 years of fol-
> low-up.

> (2007: 227–228)

These authors also suggest that the women at highest risk are those between
the ages of puberty and 30. This is particularly relevant to my participants

who fall into this age group. It is important to emphasise that recent technical advances have significantly reduced the risk of post therapy new cancers (Zablotska *et al.* 2007) and the unanticipated late effect of the early mantle field radiotherapy is not typical of any of the other cancer treatments charted in this volume. Nevertheless, I feel it is of importance to represent some instances of this experience, as the ways in which the legacy is experienced by the survivor and managed by the medical professionals can also inform us about the wider range of impacts for survivors of other cancers.

The physical legacy

The physical symptoms experienced by the participants were many and varied, some resulted in continuing pain or discomfort and had an ongoing impact on quality of life and physical ability. Others legacies did not result in impairment and carried with them no further implications for later ill health. However, the impact is not related directly to the nature of the physical legacy as Elizabeth Bryan's account of the feelings evoked by scars shows:

> The constant reminders of my cancer don't help. Take my scars: my botched appendectomy and various cuts and burns are just relics of the past of my history, not my present. But the two inelegant mastectomies and the large, but beautifully healed abdominal scar are different. They are reminders of ongoing vulnerability.
>
> (2008: 5)

Although Bryan was facing the prospect of death from an hereditary cancer which ultimately claimed her life, the meaning attached to scars became apparent amongst my participants even years after the cancer and even when death was not an expected outcome. The following quote from Gillian articulates the connection between the physical and emotional effects which suggests that the visible physical legacy can carry with it an additional meaning beyond any pain or limitation:

> I suppose in a way it makes me feel a little bit different. Yes, it just makes me feel different ... if you've had a cancer I suppose yes you feel you're never the same again ... because I had my spleen out ... I've got you know a huge big scar right down my middle. I see that every day. So it is a reminder ... I mean it's not visible to anybody else, obviously my neck is where I had a biopsy, but nothing else is visible. But it's visible to me. And that is in a way a daily reminder. I don't like that. I mean I don't like having it. They did little blue tattoos front and back – like little blue dots. And of course they're there permanently. And every time ... you know if ever I'm examined medically, you know 'Oh what are those?' Because it's surprising quite a few doctors don't know. And then you have to explain ... and other medical things, whenever I go to anything else, any clinics,

it's always you know your past history. And you're having to repeat it each time, so you're not allowed to forget it.

(Gillian: 34 yrs after diagnosis with Hodgkin's lymphoma)

Gillian does not address the medical implications of her splenectomy yet the scar clearly carries with it significant meaning that may not be apparent to others. Despite the fact that no one else can see Gillian's scar, the constant reminder every time she dresses or bathes brings with it painful memories even 34 years after she was diagnosed. The scars and the tattoos also necessitate her revisiting the illness at every medical encounter, while the tattoos might be considered trivial in contrast to having experienced a life-threatening illness, they clearly have a significant symbolic meaning and as Gillian says 'you're not allowed to forget'. Kate offered a similar account; for her even a trip to the hairdresser necessitated her explaining her scar:

I've got an enormous scar ... it's like the M1 down there ... [so] when I was young and reasonably skinny, I wouldn't have worn a bikini ... it goes from sort of basically under the ribcage, down past the belly button, down to sort of one hipbone ... it's enormous, yes. I mean it's at least a foot long I would say ... there's one on my neck, which is probably about ... three or four inches long, where I had a biopsy done ... that was where the lump was ... I'm still conscious of it. So my hair is long ... if I ever get a new hairdresser, they always say, 'Oh that's a nasty scar.' I go through the rigmarole of oh yes well I had cancer.

(Kate: 31 yrs after diagnosis with Hodgkin's lymphoma)

Both Paul, nine years after diagnosis with testicular cancer, and Linda, 28 years after diagnosis with Hodgkin's lymphoma talked of their embarrassment at the scars on their bodies. However, it seems that it is not the visible physical scars *per se* that affect confidence, it is the meaning attached to that legacy as shown in the following account by Marc who had had his leg amputated at the time of the illness. Yet this irreversible and apparently far-reaching consequence is not even mentioned in his summary – indeed towards the end he even seems to be searching for possible effects he might have overlooked.

I come from a family of people who have very thick hair, and my hair never really grew back how it was. And so I was always thinning on top, right from being 18 ... It was a mild irritation you know. I would have preferred it not to have been like that. I mean I'd prefer not to be like that now, but you know in the scheme of things, you know it was relatively small – a small price to pay. So there's that. My hearing is slightly impaired. And I think that was possibly the cysplatin that did that, one of the chemo drugs that I had ... It means that I'm not very good with background noise, so in kind of loud, busy environments that kind of can be a bit of an issue. Sorry, I'm trying to think if there's any other physical effects.

(Marc: 21 yrs after diagnosis with osteosarcoma)

While the physical evidence of Kate's and Gillian's illnesses did not appear to cause them pain or discomfort, the same cannot be said of many of other survivors. In contrast to Kate and Gillian, Meg – diagnosed with the same cancer – had endured nearly 40 years of debilitating physical symptoms that had shaped the course of her life; indeed it was only relatively recently that she had been referred to a pain clinic which appeared to be helping her:

> I was having problems swallowing ... I felt like a snake that had eaten something too big for itself ... I nearly choked on a sandwich when I was out ... I've had problems with my back aching and my shoulder aching, and the top of my neck last year ... I was under a rheumatologist for a few years ... and he sent me to see a neurologist and he suggested I should see a pain clinic then. So when I saw the rheumatologist ... he disagreed and said 'no, no, you know, you don't need to see the pain clinic'. And now he's since retired and the young consultant took over. And she said there was nothing really that she could do for me you know. So she said you know I'll just discharge you. So I asked her if I could be referred to the pain clinic. So she referred me, and I've since being going to the pain clinic. And it has helped an awful lot.
>
> (Meg: 38 yrs after diagnosis with Hodgkin's lymphoma)

It appears that Meg was not afforded easy access to the pain clinic which now seems to be alleviating her symptoms. Determination to be referred was required as the health professionals seemed either unaware of the impact of her symptoms or the benefits that could be derived from pain management intervention. But Meg's physical symptoms had a wider impact; she told me how the ongoing problems with swallowing affected her social life as she found eating out at restaurants very difficult.

Like Meg, Richard too told me of the many years of pain resulting from his cancer 36 years earlier. Having attended a number of pain clinics Richard is still searching for effective pain management, though he had accepted that ongoing pain was something he just had to learn to live with. While pain was a problem for some, others spoke of a 'general malaise' coupled with a susceptibility to infection, for example, Kelly, whose main physical legacy is extreme tiredness. For a young woman whose friends expect to party late into the night this presents not just a physical challenge but also a social one. Kelly had thought that after 6 years she should be feeling stronger and seems unable to imagine a time when she might overcome the tiredness:

> I experience quite extreme tiredness ... I've asked about it, and they don't really seem to have any suggestions about what I can do ... I've been out

with my partner when he was at university and I've either had to go home, back to his house early, or we've both had to leave early, because it gets to the early hours – even though I know I haven't got any work to do for the next few days – it gets to the early hours and I just have to go. I can't stay any longer. And then it'll take me days and days to catch up on that sleep ... it's something that I thought after 6 years would probably disappear.

(Kelly: 7 yrs after diagnosis with non-Hodgkin's lymphoma)

Greg's surgery for the osteosarcoma in his arm and the lung secondaries that followed had left him with a range of ongoing physical symptoms:

Well I like to think that I was always going to be sort of very strong, big, and I'm just ridiculously thin and I can't seem to shift that in any way ... as far as my arm's concerned I've got this restricted use of the arm ... you can look at it in two ways, you could say it affects everything, because it's slightly there in everything that I do. And at the same time it doesn't really affect anything. There's nothing major that I can't do. I think most people have it [osteosarcoma] in their leg and it was funny when we used to meet at hospital and got to know each other all, a lot of us very well. The first time we'd sort of talk about it and we'd have, me and another lad who, who had it in his leg started talking together. And we both 'oh I feel so sorry for you having it in your leg', 'oh so sorry you had it in your arm'. We'd both been indoctrinated with the positives of the way round that we had it ... I'd still probably rather have had it in the arm because there's nothing noticeable. You know you can walk around, run, you can play just about all sports. In fact the only thing they said not to do was play golf and cricket, so I started playing golf ... there's more of a worry that they tend to break I think. And mine never has. But there's almost nothing connecting it together. So when you lift stuff you, you just don't know whether it's going to go one day.

(Greg: 19 yrs after diagnosis with osteosarcoma)

Greg has an ongoing legacy of pain but has not allowed either this, or the warnings to avoid certain sports, to curtail his activities. He has learned to incorporate his physical limitations and even be thankful that the osteosarcoma was in his arm rather than his leg which he feels would have left him with greater restrictions. It may be significant that he tells us of the 'indoctrination' of being positive about the location of the osteosarcoma at the time of treatment and that this effect has been a lasting one – he has taken a 'glass half full' rather than a 'glass half empty' approach to his interpretation of how it affects his life. Greg's extreme thinness can be contrasted with the weight gain and lasting stretch marks that some survivors like Ben experience:

It changed a lot about how I looked, because when I had chemotherapy I got a lot of water retention, and I gained quite a lot of weight with water retention ... I've got a lot of stretch marks ... I've got them on my legs as well. But the worst problem I've had, and I've been to the doctors about it ... some muscles have been damaged because I have real big problems with my hip ... sometimes I have real trouble like walking on it, real sharp shooting pain in it.

(Ben: 4 yrs after diagnosis with testicular cancer)

Thomas told me that the physical legacy of his brain tumour had had a profound effect on his body image as he too had gained a considerable amount of weight because of his treatment. At one point his weight had reached 20 stone. While he had successfully managed to lose some of the weight, as with Ben, the resulting stretch marks were, he feared permanent. Thomas is the only survivor of a brain tumour included in this study. I suspect that this is in part because the physical and social consequences of a brain tumour can be so devastating that the resulting isolation lessens the likelihood of participation. However, this is only supposition on my part, whatever the reason, we have only Thomas' account of what survival after a brain tumour has meant, but it is clear that the ongoing physical impact affected Thomas' academic career badly; the impact on life plans is a theme developed more fully in Chapter 7:

It has presented me with some things that are difficult, challenging, and a lot of sadness I think in my life. I mean [I] take a conglomerate of pills everyday ... I have to do a great hormone injection ... one of the biggest problems is that I seem to be something of a kleptomaniac when it comes to illness ... the sequel of the cancer has sort of rolled on through my life, and it's taken me out ... I managed to get to Bristol Uni, but then had to drop out for a year because I had a problem with illness. And then I went back to try again, but I was desperately ill with seizures – brain stem seizures, not epileptic seizures – resulting from where the second tumour was on the cerebellum, the brain stem. And that took me out of the university completely. And I used to spend a lot of time in the hospital ... I developed diabetes as well.

(Thomas: 13 yrs after diagnosis with a brain tumour)

There is evidence in these accounts of the physical legacy that there can be an accompanying emotional and social impact, but this is writ large with Maz whose entire life seems to have been negatively affected by the physical legacy:

I just feel so ... you know like, can't survive, like really difficult to manage everything because I'm just alone myself ... I got sexual problems, I've got mobility problems ... and that's why I'm just a bit upset about myself ... I'm seeing loads of people, they are suffering after the treatment also. And I'm one of them you see ... I can't walk normally because they've taken all my bones, and my pelvis ... I go limping along all the time. And that's why I can't do jobs because I can't pick the heavy stuff up, I can't sit down very long because my back is hurting ... I can't do any jobs ... sometimes I'm so ill, sometimes I've got so much pain in my leg ... always but sometimes it's worse, especially on the cold days it's worse ... Really I don't know myself. That's why I'm just confused. I'm totally confused ... I'm losing my speech ... I'm losing my memory, totally lost my memory. I can't remember your name ... can't remember anything you know.

> (Maz: 4 yrs after diagnosis with Ewing's sarcoma)

While John's physical legacy may not be as debilitating, he has nevertheless had to manage a number of late effects. He was one of many of the lymphoma survivors who spoke of thyroid problems, but in addition he expressed concern about the long-term effects of radiotherapy:

I currently have an underactive thyroid gland. I have an underactive pituitary gland. Because of the underactive pituitary – I have to take a hormone injection every 8 weeks, it's not pleasant. Again, although no one can say for certain, I had a polyp removed last year, which was potentially as a result of the chemotherapy. I've just recently discovered that I have a rare type of basal cell on my tummy, which has got to be surgically removed in a couple of weeks. Again that was in the field of the radiotherapy.

> (John: 33 yrs after diagnosis with Hodgkin's lymphoma)

Another survivor of Hodgkin's lymphoma, Debbie, said that the physical legacy had been with her for more than 20 years and even relatively trivial consequences, such as having to be careful what flavour crisps to eat, acted as continuing daily reminders of the illness:

I've got to be honest, there probably isn't a day that goes by when I don't think about the treatment or the lymphoma ... because it still impacts on my life quite a lot ... I've still got reduced salivary flow. My mouth is fairly sensitive still to ... you know I can't eat fresh pineapple, I'm not very good with citrus fruit, salt and vinegar crisps are no good, you know very spicy food. So I have to you know, watch what I eat sort of thing ... I get a lot of sore throats because I'm still quite dry ... I've got very marked muscle fibrosis in my neck and shoulders ... that's apparently from the radiotherapy.

> (Debbie: 22 yrs after diagnosis with Hodgkin's lymphoma)

Gillian, another long-term Hodgkin's lymphoma survivor, also had a thyroid problem but in addition told me of her early menopause:

After about ten years the thyroid packed up. And I did go through an early menopause age 36 ... a couple of weeks ago I went to see a gynaecologist, and he said oh well of course you know these problems that you're having at the moment, it's probably all because you went through the early menopause. And I think well ... so there is a knock on effect yes ... I did have my spleen out. And a lot obviously [of] infections ... this time last year I did have quite severe pneumonia ... my GP [says] 'well you know, you haven't got the defences, you haven't got ... look at your history'.

(Gillian: 34 yrs after diagnosis with Hodgkin's lymphoma)

Gillian's early menopause is clearly a concern to young women who have not yet had children and is an issue that is elaborated on in Chapter 8. The ongoing physical problems from the effect on Kate's spleen and thyroid are still of active concern to her 13 years later and like Gillian she is vulnerable to pneumonia and other infections which could be potentially fatal if not caught early:

I do have long-term side effects from the treatment which I received. I had my spleen removed, so I've got very low immunity to certain types of bacteria. And I also had radiotherapy to the glands that were affected, which were in the neck, so my thyroid gland was destroyed. So I've got an underactive thyroid gland. So I have to put up with those, and you know this is life-long. And I have to be quite careful, and I have to make sure I ... you know if I get sick with like pneumonia I have to really go to the doctor's very quickly because it's fatal in five hours.

(Kate: 31 yrs after diagnosis with Hodgkin's lymphoma)

For Elaine B the heart trouble she has been left with is an ongoing concern in addition to her thyroid problems:

I do have problems with my heart, because of the chemotherapy boost on it ... they actually found a hole in my heart, but they said that could have been there from being born ... but I have got a floppy mitral value ... chemotherapy does weaken the heart valves ... I am on Beta Blockers because my heart beat is a bit too fast. But that's only since last year when I fell in the bath, and broke my ribs ... It shook my heart rate up, so they put me on Beta Blockers – only since last year ... I go for a mammogram check-up every year. And so far – touch wood – everything's been clear there. That's because I had radiotherapy to my chest. They check on that, and every year ... but that's good ... they took half my thyroid because there was a goitre ... So they took half of it out, and luckily that came back as benign.

(Elaine B: 15 yrs after diagnosis with Hodgkin's lymphoma)

We have seen that a number of the lymphoma survivors experience thyroid problems yet it seems that not only had Julie been unprepared for the possibility that her thyroid might be affected, her GP was also unaware of the link. It was only because of finding information provided by the Lymphoma Association that Julie was able to alert her doctor to the connection:

> And it was because of reading that [the Lymphoma Association newsletter], I later found out that I had a thyroid problem I didn't ... because I didn't realise, [that] another kind of one of these knock on effects of having the radiotherapy is that, after 5 years it's possible for your thyroid to start to fail. And it comes on gradually, and you just kind of ... you don't notice it at first, and you just think you're feeling a bit down. But reading this ... they said, oh these are the symptoms – failing thyroid. Oh I thought, oh my goodness. These are all the things I've been having. I had a test at the doctors, and yes, it was failing.
>
> No, I know definitely it wouldn't have [been picked up without that information] because I had to take it up with the oncologist. And because they just didn't test thyroid function at all, even though there was this study out to say yes definitely, thyroid function's affected – or can be affected ... So I said you need to test this. You need to be checking all your patients who've had that kind of radiotherapy, after 5 years. And he wouldn't believe me at first, but he wrote off to Christies for advice, and they said 'you should be doing this, why aren't you?' So I felt quite pleased about that, because I thought well that's good, because that's helped people.
>
> (Julie: 15 yrs after first diagnosis with Hodgkin's lymphoma)

It seems surprising given the number of participants who had thyroid problems resulting from Hodgkin's lymphoma that Julie's GP was unaware of the relationship and apparently needed to be convinced that this was a problem. Thus it appears that GPs may find it difficult to keep up to date with the latest research and information on late effects.

There were many other examples of lasting physical effects, several participants told me that because of the high number of blood transfusions they had had during the cancer treatment, they now had to have blood drawn on a regular basis to bring down a potentially damaging iron count. Again such an effect while not necessarily serious, debilitating or a cause of anxiety nevertheless was a continuing reminder even many years later. As Rowena said having to go in six times a year for this treatment meant that she could not leave the illness behind her:

> You want to get back to your normality and you can't quite do that. And I don't think you ever will quite do that.
>
> (Rowena: 12 yrs after first diagnosis with Hodgkin's lymphoma)

Fifteen years after Julie had been diagnosed with Hodgkin's lymphoma she was diagnosed with breast cancer that was a direct result of the mantle field radiotherapy she had received 14 years earlier. She was not angry or resentful that her treatment had caused breast cancer, what she was angry about was that she had chanced upon the study that suggested she was at risk, but she was unable to secure an early mammogram or preventative elective treatment to limit the chances of her developing the illness. Despite repeated visits to her GP, her oncologist and a failed attempt to pay for a private mammogram; by the time she was referred for the screening test she had already developed breast cancer. Julie felt angry that her anxieties had been dismissed by professionals as 'neurotic' and that as a result she had needed a mastectomy. At the time of my interview with her she was planning a second elective mastectomy as she was afraid of developing cancer in her remaining breast. In addition to a thyroid condition, Julie had some mobility problems which she said had been exacerbated by the cancer:

> I've always had weight problems [but they've been] made worse ... and I've got a long-term back problem since I've had the chemo ... your level of fitness goes like ... it's amazing how long it takes for you to feel strong you know, because it's like you're physically feel weak – I can't describe it ... And then when you want to do things, it sort of ... the energy just isn't there. The power isn't there you know. You want to lift something and it's just you think ... Yes, I can't lift that. I can normally just do it, and it's like a kettle! And just ridiculous things ... I find it a bit kind of upsetting sometimes that I can't go and enjoy walks and you know, sort of things we used to do ... there was a lot of family experiences, days out, going places you know, that has just not really been possible you know.
> (Julie: 15 yrs after first diagnosis with Hodgkin's lymphoma)

Mary too had been diagnosed with treatment-related breast cancer and, like Julie, she also feels that she was failed. Despite the fact that in her case she had been offered mammography, this was not sufficient to pick up her breast cancer at an early stage:

> I actually think the late effects follow-up is poor in areas ... I went for lots of investigation – mammography and MRIs, and at that point I'd just got married again for the second time. And I was sort of rejoicing in being fit, healthy, alive, sexy ... thinking I might try for a family very soon. I did not want to have a double mastectomy. No. And I decided I'd go for the long-term monitoring instead. And now in fact the monitoring has let me down, because my cancer wasn't actually picked up on the MRI scan ... it's not terribly effective on women under 40 ... because I've quite small, dense breasts – I haven't had any children. It's not very good at picking them up. You know I didn't quite realise that. Well even my husband who's a GP didn't realise that. And also I think I'd always thought well if I do get the breast cancer it'll be caught early. Actually it wasn't caught very early, and also unfortunately mine's a grade 3. And I didn't realise

there were different grades. I thought you got breast cancer and you just got the lump out, and a bit of radiotherapy. I didn't realise I couldn't have any more radiotherapy because I've had so much before. So my treatment now for breast cancer is very much compromised by what I've had before, which wasn't explained to me ... In fact both of the lymphoma follow-up clinics who have followed me up actually are both kicking themselves, and are very, very sorry, and have apologised to me that they didn't examine my breasts ... checking me up, you know all my lymph sites, they've been taking a blood test off me, but nobody's been doing a breast examination or checking that I was doing one properly ... It's been very much sort of you're in the late effects clinic, this, this, and this is relevant. They really want to pat you on your head. In fact at my ... appointment which was September 13th this year, at [the] Hospital, they interviewed me and photographed me as a long-term successful survivor, and actually published me in their Christmas appeal – but failed to examine my breasts ... so busy telling me what a great survivor I was ... I'm angry, boy am I angry! I'm seriously angry. I'm not angry that I've got it, because I can accept that that's a hazard of medicine. You know what I was treated with at 24 was the state of the art treatment, it's still a treatment now, although slightly modified. And that's just a hazard of radiotherapy. And I've had 20 very good years, but nonetheless my follow-up and screening process have actually let me down, unfortunately. You know it wouldn't have stopped me getting it, but it might have caught it a bit earlier. It might not have actually spread.

(Mary: 24 yrs after diagnosis with Hodgkin's lymphoma)

There is an extended discussion of long-term follow-up clinics in the next chapter, but suffice it to say here that the reassurance that long-term monitoring should give patients, in Mary's case, appears to have let her down. Like Julie, Mary is angry, not because of the second treatment-related cancer, but because of what she perceives to be the mishandling of her follow-up. She also specifies the issue of life cycle and the need for clinicians to recognise that the late effects of cancer in young adulthood carry long-term wider implications not only, for the life stage effects of planning of pregnancy, but also the diagnostic implications of the nature of breast tissue in this age group. It also seems that the celebration of her 'successful survivorship' may have obscured her need for further investigation.

Linda had also had Hodgkin's lymphoma 28 years before she spoke to me. Although she had had follow-up appointments for 10 years after the illness, during the intervening period with no follow-up to remind her on a regular basis, she had tried to put her illness history to the back of her mind – but then she had a letter calling her to attend the breast clinic and was catapulted back emotionally to her earlier cancer experience. She said she felt panic but had no one to talk to about it. This suggests that under such circumstances a personal approach that offers information and support would be a more sensitive way to manage the situation. Linda would clearly have welcomed the chance to discuss this new threat to her health caused by her earlier treatment but had not been given the opportunity. Like Julie, Mary and Linda, Lesley had undergone treatment for Hodgkin's lymphoma, in her case 18 years earlier, that could have increased her chances of getting breast cancer. Like Linda she had been unprepared for the shock when she received the call for a mammogram. Lesley had been for three mammograms and told me how anxious she became before each recall.

It is clear that there are a range of lasting physical effects that are interpreted and experienced in different ways. The negative meaning attributed to scarring or tattoos or stretch marks – none of which are indicative of any ongoing threat to health – may seem unexpected. Such scars could be interpreted as 'heroic' yet if we remember the age group, and how important body image is to them, the negative reaction becomes less surprising. But there is also evidence that survivors can experience non serious symptoms that they perceive as threatening of future illness or malignancy. Even for some of those who do not manifest sinister symptoms there were indications of a continuing and sometimes increasing anxiety about their health. It is to this issue that we now turn.

Ongoing anxiety

According to McKenzie and Crouch (2004) once the diagnosis, treatment and immediate aftermath are past, the 'struggle' is deemed to be over. This may mean an expectation from self and others that life should continue as before, and that the survivor should move on with their lives and return to what McKenzie and Crouch describe as an 'even keel' (2004: 144). Yet it is clear from the accounts provided earlier that there are a range of late effects and physical consequences of the illness and its treatment that may make such a return to 'normality' difficult and there are also indications that there may be fears of a relapse. We have already seen the anxiety caused to the female Hodgkin's lymphoma survivors who had been warned of their increased risk of breast cancer. But even in the absence of such explicit warnings survivors may carry with them an underlying fear of recurrence.

According to Langeveld and Arbuckle the fear of relapse can be a major anxiety for a considerable period after treatment is over. As these authors say 'aches and pains that they previously shrugged off now contribute to a fear of the cancer returning' (2008: 155–156). This is evidenced earlier as some of the late effects we have seen documented could be feared to herald the return of the cancer or the development of a second treatment-related cancer. This raises the question of how such concerns are, or should be, managed and how they impact on the quality of survivorship.

Many survivors will turn to their GP for support and advice, but we have already seen in some of the earlier accounts that GPs are not always up to date with the most recent studies on late effects. This may not be surprising as according to Oeffinger:

> Many physicians feel overwhelmed by the new information in this field and by the relative lack of composite or general resources available to clinicians and scientists who provide health care to cancer survivors or investigate their health problems and needs.
>
> (2007: 2209)

Yet because of a combination of late effects and anxieties, that may or may not relate to any identifiable physical symptom, survivors need recourse to reliable advice. In his professional role as a cancer nurse, John made the following remark based on his own survivorship experience and also upon the observations of his patients:

> In my opinion … once diagnosed with a cancer … it's a life-long legacy that never leaves you. I think … that has been borne out by many patients today who maybe have aches and pains, or you know a cold, coughs, and different ailments. And they automatically think is this the cancer making an unheralded return. On one occasion I was having these splitting headaches for no apparent reason, just searing headaches … those proved to be some form of migraine ice-pick headaches. Again you know the fear was, was this returning? This was some 21, 22 years after diagnosis. So it's always in the back of the mind.
>
> (John: 33 yrs after diagnosis with Hodgkin's lymphoma)

John's use of the term 'life-long legacy' was echoed by others and is illustrated well by Lesley who speaks of her inability to leave the cancer in the past:

> I think as a cancer survivor your biggest fear is it reoccurring. So there is always that in the back of your mind … I had a bit of a scare with my back I had a bleed in my spine … I just immediately thought 'oh here we go again' … that is your biggest fear … I do feel sometimes like I passed that 10 year milestone of being signed off, but every now and again I just get a bit of a slap round the face and it reminds me, and it's sort of back with me. You know that I can never sort of totally put it behind me.
>
> (Lesley: 18 yrs after diagnosis with Hodgkin's lymphoma)

Debbie too had been recalled for breast screening but her account shows the extent of her anxieties beyond breast cancer and like Lesley she specifies the significance of the '10 year milestone' and her disappointment that the 'all clear' and the resulting release from further concern seemed to be an ever receding likelihood:

> To be honest, I think in the beginning it was sort of getting to the 10 year mark. And then everything was going to be fantastic. And then recently,

because there appears to be more and more long-term side effects that they're now discovering, it's quite a feeling of uncertainty sometimes I have to say. For instance I'm part of the programme at Guy's where I now have to go and have an annual mammogram. And I see the breast clinic, because of the increased risk of breast cancer. There's obviously the increased risk of lung cancer and skin cancer as well. My thyroid's inactive. I'm on thyroxine now, which they think is a result of that. And I think sort of, for me, having gone for so many years and, wow you're a real success, this is fantastic, de, de, de, de, de ... you know it's really great – quite often when I go now there's almost like a little bit of bad news each time. So ... which I find emotionally sets me back a little bit for a few days ... when all the hooh-hah hit about the breast cancer and everything ... of course, you know it was in the papers, and it was all over the website and I was sort of reading it – and I'm a very level-headed sort of person, and I knew that it would be discussed at my next appointment and everything – but where there was ... on the lymphoma website there was a list of – I don't know – five high risk factors, and I ticked the box for four of them. And it just made me feel vulnerable again.

(Debbie: 22 yrs after diagnosis with Hodgkin's lymphoma)

Debbie describes herself as 'vulnerable' and there are indications in the quotation later that Kelly too feels a similar vulnerability. However Kelly, whose family had a tendency not to go to the doctors and whose upbringing did not encourage the sick role, uses the term 'paranoid' when expressing her concerns about symptoms that could herald a relapse:

My cancer wasn't colon cancer, but it presented around the colon. And if I have any pains at all in that area at all, I get quite paranoid. Most of the time I'll give it a few days, and if it disappears I won't do anything about it. But I have rung the GP about it and been down to see her before, I have rung my consultant on a couple of occasions and just said I'm worried about this. And that's something that I would never have done, because I come from a family who don't go to the doctor about anything. You know from parents who were teachers, who took you into school and only left you at home if you were actually being sick.

(Kelly: 7 yrs after diagnosis with non-Hodgkin's lymphoma)

The recall for breast screening experienced by the women survivors of lymphoma generated a considerable amount of very understandable anxiety. However, as Janet tells us, her anxiety predated the recall and had been an increasing phenomenon:

I've worried more and more, different phases in my life – particularly when I got married, could I have children? and things like that. And now in actual fact, I am being told now that [because of] the treatment I had

that I'm at a high risk for getting breast cancer now because of the radiotherapy I received. So that's another worry now really.

> (Janet: 27 yrs after diagnosis with Hodgkin's lymphoma)

Even before Julie knew that the treatment she had received for Hodgkin's
lymphoma was likely to put her at risk from breast cancer she, like Janet, had
worried about a late and serious implication:

> Oh I did [worry] ... my fear was if it was [if it] did return, I knew that it
> would be a more serious matter. And that was always something that
> would be at the back of my mind. So I hadn't actually worried about the
> first bout, but it was the thought of having something more serious, did
> worry me.
>
> (Julie: 15 yrs after first diagnosis with Hodgkin's lymphoma)

Julie's later mastectomy for breast cancer and planned elective mastectomy of
her remaining breast should have eased her concerns, but she pointed out that
without breasts no mammography was possible though some breast tissue
might remain and put her at ongoing risk:

> I know the chances of the cancer returning after the mastectomy goes
> down like 90 per cent or something like that – and that's brilliant. But
> going back to ... revisiting the thing about like being discharged from the
> hospital and everything, there then becomes a point well you can't have
> the mammogram then ... [but] how do I know there's not anything going
> on ... because you still have breast tissue ... and it comes down to the
> point well all you can do is just check manually. And that comes down to
> yourself you know, really.
>
> (Julie: 15 yrs after first diagnosis with Hodgkin's lymphoma)

Rowena was also one of the survivors at increased risk of breast cancer, but
in addition to this concern she also worried about relatively minor symptoms
lest they should herald a recurrence. Given that she developed a second
cancer 4 years after the first, this puts her concern into some context:

> I do [worry] with a cough because that's how it got first diagnosed. I had
> this cough and I couldn't get rid of it. I think it makes you more of a
> hypochondriac maybe ... it's always in the back of mind. Not so much as
> it used to be, but it is always there. So when you do fall ill, or when you
> feel tired, or you know out of breath or something, which are all the
> symptoms I had right from the start, you kind of think oh, what if it's
> come back. You know deep down that you feel fine, and you know deep
> down that it probably isn't, but it's always there, just that slight little 1
> per cent in your mind going, 'What if?' I mean I'm the sort of person
> that's never asked the question, you know what if it did come back again?

You know would there be any options left open for me because of the three things that I've been through if you like. You kind of think would that be the end of the road. But I've never wanted to ask that question because I don't want to know the answer. As long as I feel fine I kind of try and bury my head and say I'm fine. And until that happens I'm not going to ask the questions. Or if it happens – hopefully it won't but ...

(Rowena: 12 yrs after first diagnosis with Hodgkin's lymphoma)

It is interesting that here Rowena says that she has chosen 'not to ask the questions', she also told me that she would not have wanted to know at the point of diagnosis all the longer-term effects and that to cope with each episode or challenge as and when it occurred was as much as she could deal with. Mary too had been diagnosed with a treatment-related breast cancer but talked about how her hatred of being a patient had been in ascendency over her tendency to hypochondria, meaning that she never visited the doctor if she could avoid it even though she worried about her health.

Louise had been diagnosed with a kidney problem after her cancer, but her doctors disagreed about whether it had been caused by her treatment. Whether or not this additional health concern was related, she bundled all her symptoms together and worried generally about her health:

I've got like a chunk missing out my back now where they took the muscle out. And sometimes when I get like aches there ... it's normal for me to worry. And obviously I do worry because I've got like high blood pressure as well. And that ... obviously that links with the kidney ... function. It just means though ... I do worry about things, yes.

(Louise: 8 yrs after diagnosis with Ewing's sarcoma)

There appeared amongst some participants to be an underlying belief that genetic tendencies or links are powerful and inescapable. Linda clearly perceives herself to be at risk genetically and that this is a physiological tendency she cannot avoid:

Yes. I think ... if you have that particular gene in your body anyway it's there. And I think maybe, you know it'll come back. That's my biggest fear really ... I mean that's always sort of been there in the back of my mind, that I've had it once, it might come back.

(Linda: 28 yrs after diagnosis with Hodgkin's lymphoma)

For some of the women participants, the genetic aspects of the illness extended their concern to that of the health of their children and even to their grandchildren; and it may be significant that no male participants addressed this issue as a concern. Lesley had an underlying anxiety over her children's health that was manifested in a fear that her daughter might be infertile as a result of her cancer. Interestingly this concern did not extend to her son's fertility though Lesley acknowledged that this was not necessarily rational:

> [I] ... do sometimes ... wonder if Jade will be able to conceive naturally. I don't know where that comes from ... I don't ... think that it's hereditary in any way, because I'm sure I've been told it isn't.
> (Lesley: 18 yrs after diagnosis with Hodgkin's lymphoma)

Janet also appeared to be more concerned for her daughter's health than for her own. She told me that a problem with her daughter's lymph glands in her groin resulted in one of her legs being affected by a distressing lymphoedema.

> Funnily enough my daughter was actually born with a condition which is ... it's a problem with her lymph glands as well, although they do assure me it's completely coincidental.
> (Janet: 27 yrs after diagnosis with Hodgkin's lymphoma)

Although Janet had been assured that there was no connection to her lymphoma, she could not help but connect the two lymphatic conditions and felt that the lymphatic condition her daughter had been born with might have some connection to her own lymphoma. Similar to Katie's concern that her son's Cystic Fibrosis might be connected to her cancer (see Chapter 8), Janet spoke of the guilt she would feel if her own illness had caused her daughter's condition. Despite the fact that Gillian's children and grandchild had not had health problems she too was worried her cancer history might have affected them:

> But nobody could tell me anything ... I'd like to know now ... I mean my children ... I'd like to know if they are at any higher risk, because I had it ... but ditto my grandchild – is she going to be higher risk?
> (Gillian: 34 yrs after diagnosis with Hodgkin's lymphoma)

Thus it seems that for those women who do give birth there may be a tendency to link any illnesses in their children to their own cancers, and worry for their well-being even if they are not ill and even if they are assured by health professionals that there is no risk.

Quentin has lived with the underlying concern that his treatment, more than 30 years earlier, might still be the cause of a future cancer-related illness and has taken the stance that should this be the case he would refuse further treatment.

> I've often considered over the years, that radiotherapy was pretty intense. And if you think about back to 1974 then probably the dosages were high by modern standards, that if there was going to be a long-term consequence ... it would be as a result of being subjected to something like the

equivalent of Hiroshima. In the end I might develop cancer, ironically enough, as a result of the radiotherapy. It wouldn't surprise me in the slightest, and I've always known that, and I've always considered it as a possibility ... I had to go and have my wisdom teeth out in the late 1980s ... in fact the dentist suggested to me that the bone structure – my jaw and so on – had been affected by the radiation ... subsequently I've always held in my mind the possibility that, you know it might have a deleterious effect on me at some point in time ... I've always told myself ... that if I ever got cancer again, that given my experience of the treatment last time, and given what I know about the treatment of cancer in terms of chemotherapy, which I did not have, that I would actually refuse to have treatment ... you know that I wasn't going to go through that again because ... this time it would be different ... there's no way I would want to go through radical radiotherapy, surgery, chemotherapy, you know in order only to die in the end anyway from the disease ... I could not be doing with doing it again you know ... once is enough. The logic is this ... should the radiotherapy have that effect ... it'll probably be terminal ... it will be an unusual and unpleasant form of cancer, and I don't wish to bother with treating it.

(Quentin: 33 yrs after diagnosis with Hodgkin's lymphoma)

A few weeks after I had interviewed Quentin he became unwell with breathing difficulties. As soon as he sought medical advice it was clear that once the professionals had seen 'lymphoma' in his medical history they were concerned about a possible link. After several weeks, having seen consultants from different specialisms, but with no definitive diagnosis, the symptoms gradually subsided. Clearly such an episode would generate anxiety in a person with no cancer history, but where there is a history it is understandable that the survivor's thoughts turn to the possibility of the illness being cancer related. Even though Paul B's heavy cold and cough was not as serious potentially as Quentin's breathing problems, he still spoke of how easy it was to attribute a relatively routine illness to a recurrence:

That's the worst time ... I've had one [a cough] just recently ... I've had a bit of a heavy cold, and ended up with a bit of a chest infection ... it didn't seem to be shifting ... you start thinking then ... now every time I get a cough and it's lasting longer than a week I'm thinking, hang on ... this time I was thinking Christ, hang on it's not going ... I think that's something I'll always ... have in the back of my mind now ... if you have any of the [original] symptoms you do sort of think ... I hope this isn't anything a bit more sinister than it probably is ... that's definitely something you do always ... you always have in the back of your mind.

(Paul B: 11 yrs after diagnosis with non-Hodgkin's lymphoma)

'Always have in the back of your mind' is reminiscent of Quentin's reflections and suggests a tendency to live with a low grade underlying concern.

However, Majad's anxiety and fear of relapse appeared to be a constant concern at the forefront of his mind:

> You know because it's always in my head isn't it. I'm thinking in my head, you know is it going to come back, is it not going to come back, or what's going to happen? It's always in my head you know. But I know for sure now, you know fingers crossed, you know that it's not going to come back. Well I hope it doesn't anyway. You know, but it's just always in my head. It's always in the back of my head thinking 'oh no'.
>
> (Majad: 7 yrs after diagnosis with testicular cancer)

Rizwana, Majad's wife was present at the interview and said:

> Anything just triggers him off ... stomach pain or anything and he's always going 'oh no it could be, it could be, it could be'. And then he puts me down because it's like 'oh no'. You know he's thinking like that, he's making me think like that. And then it's just like stressful, really stressful ... He's like 'oh I can't ... I've got a stomach pain, I can't do this' ... he'll be in bed for days, worrying that you know it might have come back to him, and upset.
>
> (Rizwana: Majad's wife)

Clearly Majad's tendency to assume any, probably minor, ailment signalled a recurrence was affecting his family life – but he was not alone in his anxiety. Like Majad, Elaine B was concerned about what might appear to be trivial symptoms, and she, like Paul B, singled out a persistent cough as particularly worrying as this had heralded the original cancer:

> Well just recently there's been a virus hasn't there? And I'm coughing and when you're coughing you start thinking 'gosh, this is how it started first' ... you know you think 'oh is this cough going to be ... is it letting me know there's ...'? When I've got a normal cold or anything like that, I'm fine. But just coughing constantly, you start ... Well you do start to worry ... I mean you pretty much carry on with your life as normal, just sometimes checking yourself for lumps and bumps, and you just think 'oh what's that, oh no it's nothing'. You know you do ... you start feeling or thinking oh you're not well, or ... if you've got a stomach cramp, have you got stomach cramps or ... just silly little things.
>
> (Elaine B: 15 yrs after first diagnosis with Hodgkin's lymphoma)

Elaine B refers to concerns about 'silly little things' and Jamie uses the term 'paranoia' to describe the tendency to worry about 'the smallest little thing'. A number of the young men who had survived testicular cancer had learned to come to terms with living with only one testicle but the fear of a recurrence continued to cause them fear and anxiety thus a seemingly 'little thing' could have huge implications.

It's all like the smallest little thing, you sort of like well … 'could that be sort of like a side effect of that, or could it be a case of I've got cancer in a different place?' So it does make you paranoid … the thing that I'm most paranoid about is if the testicular cancer actually came back. That's the main thing that bothers me, because I mean … at the moment I've got one [testicle] so I'm alright with one … that's what the doctor said but if it comes back it just … I don't know it just …

(Jamie: 2 yrs after diagnosis with testicular cancer)

In the first chapter I recalled that in my previous study Steven had talked about feeling his neck for lumps, Kirsty echoed these words almost exactly:

When it comes to anything sort of that's related to my glands … [I'm] for-ever checking my neck where I know my tumours were. Just to make sure … before I got lymphoma I was teaching dancing, and I led quite a healthy life. And I think to me it was a bit of a shock. And probably, you know people around me thinking gosh you know. And it is true, you know anyone can get it. And it definitely made me think oh you know it's there, anything can kind of creep up on you … the thought that well if it can happen to me it can happen to anyone, and it can happen to me again … there's always that you know, niggle in the back of your head about the whole immune system and everything like that … whenever I do get ill … I think 'oh God', you know.

(Kirsty: 5 yrs after diagnosis with Hodgkin's lymphoma)

We have heard that a number of the survivors have had ongoing pain, but according to Katie pain is not the most sinister of symptoms:

I think in your mind having had it once you think it could happen. You know it's just the fact something has happened you always think well that could happen or this could happen or the other could happen … Early on particularly … I was a bit of a hypochondriac whenever I got odd pains I couldn't explain. I kept thinking is [it] there, because I hadn't got much pain the first time … it was the benign cyst that was giving me the pain the cancerous cyst hadn't given me any pain so that was always a concern that it was almost only by chance … there was always a slight concern that [there] could … be something and I wouldn't know about it … I don't think it particularly bothers me. I think well, you know they must have let me go, there must be a good reason why they don't bother monitoring me anymore … But generally on the whole I sort of trust the medical establishment to do the best within their knowledge.

(Katie: 13 yrs after diagnosis with ovarian cancer)

This response differs from Julie's in that Katie appears to have faith in the medical establishment while Julie trusts no one. These two contrasting attitudes clearly stem from experiences which either reinforce or undermine trust. Nevertheless, Katie's reluctance to undergo even routine medical procedures is clear in the following quote and is strikingly similar to Mary's resistance to undergoing fertility treatment (see Chapter 8):

> It's a little quirky thing, but for years and years I didn't want to have a smear test. Which is partly me being a bit of a chicken because I had one as part of the general diagnosis when they were working out what was wrong with me. And it hurt that much I never wanted to have another one … it was strange because at the same time I was kind of concerned that oh there could be something I wouldn't know about … but certainly in my early twenties it was almost a case of I didn't want to get bad news. So one side of me was kind of worrying, the other side of me was thinking 'but I don't want bad news and I don't want to be in hospital again and I don't want to go through it all again'.
>
> (Katie: 13 yrs after diagnosis with ovarian cancer)

While many of the accounts show how continued, low level anxiety lies just under the surface perhaps for decades, Dan suggests that the 'all clear' might be illusory and so for him it is better to accept the possibility of a recurrence:

> Okay so I survived testicular cancer … but … I don't like this idea of the 'all clear'. I think it's important psychologically for me to think that it could possibly come back. You know it's not gone … [but] I'm not completely cured if you like … yes I'm a survivor but there's nothing to say that I couldn't get something like that, or the very same again … clearly I would hate to be ill again I really would. And certainly second time round, you know that's something that I would not like at all because it's meant to be worse second time round.
>
> (Dan: 5 yrs after diagnosis with testicular cancer)

Preparation for late effects

We can see from the accounts presented thus far in this chapter that not only are there a myriad of physical legacies, they are accompanied by anxiety and concern about present and future health. Because of the age at which the cancer has been experienced, these late effects – both the actual physical impact and the concern about it – may continue for decades. This raises the question of whether there are effective ways in which survivors could be prepared for managing these ongoing manifestations of their cancer experience. Is it better to know every possible negative effect even though such effects may not be experienced by all patients – or is it better to be informed on a 'need to know' basis so that the demanding treatments can be endured without the fear that the outcome could still be a life permeated by pain and discomfort? Maz was clear and emphatic in his opinion:

I want to say a message [to professionals] ... whenever you got your patient, you have to tell everything to your patient, don't hide anything ... you got to know side effects or stuff like that, [if you don't] then you feel really hurt inside you see ... you know you have to tell him straight, you have to tell your patient straight 'this ... may affect your life and your future'. [But] they still hide stuff ... you didn't tell me this, you didn't tell me that ... you have to tell about everything ... but ... they're never telling the complete diagnosis. What happening in your future, what happening next to you and stuff like that, never been told about that ... they already know, they already know.

(Maz: 4 yrs after diagnosis with Ewing's sarcoma)

Maz appears to feel betrayed by those who cared for him, he believes they knew what he would face and deliberately withheld that information so that he has been unprepared for the many physical and emotional difficulties he now faces. In contrast, John, now a nurse of many years standing, told me that had he been warned of all the possible physical consequences of his cancer when diagnosed at the age of 18 he would not have understood the implications. Nevertheless he acknowledged that the world has changed beyond recognition in the time since his diagnosis:

There is that wonderful medium out there, the Internet, if you don't tell patients then they're going to go and find that information themselves. So I think we've got to be completely honest and sincere with patients, and we've got to tell them about you know the risks of carcinogenesis, the risks to their endocrine system, and all of the other long-term sequelae, and then allow them to make an informed decision and consent to treatment.

(John: 33 yrs after diagnosis with Hodgkin's lymphoma)

But Meg, who had experienced a range of physical difficulties resulting from her illness and treatment, said that she had had no warning that this might be the case and had just been left to 'stumble on'. Had she been prepared she said she would have felt better able to understand what was happening and why, and that this might have helped her to cope better. Gillian had lived for more than 30 years with unresolved anxieties, and even though she was still in follow up she felt unready for what survivorship would entail:

At the time I knew nothing, nobody could tell me about long-term survivorship. That is the one thing that still sticks in my mind that I would have liked to have known at the time. Of course they couldn't tell me ... was I going through all that treatment just for a few years, or for 20 years, 30 years [of life]. And the only answer I ever got was, 'we're doing this treatment, we're keeping you alive, we can't tell you anymore than that' ... I was nursing at the time ... and I have to say the only people I had ever nursed with Hodgkin's had died and I honestly thought that's what I was going to do ... it did reoccur ... I think after it reoccurred ... after the first time ... it would have been nice to know this was just a one off possibly. But nobody could tell me anything ... and I think at the time that would have been ... very important to me, to give me ... a straw to clutch onto as it were, that you know it's worth [it].

(Gillian: 34 yrs after diagnosis with Hodgkin's lymphoma)

Gillian told me that she would have been reassured to know that her resulting quality of life made the treatment worthwhile and her use of the phrase 'a straw to clutch onto' speaks volumes, but this raises the question about what those whose prognoses may be more bleak should be told when there may not be a substantial 'straw to clutch onto'. A poor prognosis may not help to prepare the survivor, Linda had been unprepared for her recall after a 20-year gap since her follow-up had finished. However, she thought that to have been pre-warned would have made that intervening period one of anxiety. Thus she believed, unlike Maz, that it was better to remain unaware of the possible consequences:

It was such a shock at the time ... because I hadn't really realised ... [but if I'd known] ... I probably would have worried about it.

(Linda: 28 yrs after diagnosis with Hodgkin's lymphoma)

The difference between Linda and Maz may in part be explained by the fact that Maz believed that his health care team had known what he would face, yet were apparently unwilling to warn him. In contrast Linda knew that the long-term effects of her radiotherapy had not been discovered until a considerable time after her treatment. This suggests that trust is central to the relationship between doctor and patient, and that it can be carried forward into future medical encounters which are shaped by previous experience. Helen had already told me she had a problem with trust and the following revelation goes some way to explaining why:

I think with regards to the doctors, they have to be aware of what they're saying to people ... particularly when you're a teenager ... some of the doctors I don't think they realise when they make comments sometimes how much that'll impact ... They're ... consultants and you're going to listen to what they say ... they didn't actually tell me I had cancer. I don't know if I was in denial, but it took 3 months and then somebody said the word ... I'd already been having chemo I had to go home to my mum and say 'have I got cancer?' And she went 'yes, didn't you realise?' Because nobody had actually told me, they just called it Hodgkin's lymphoma ... nobody really explained to me how serious it was ... nobody really explained to me the implications of that. And that you know, this was quite serious and I could die ... I think if somebody had actually not treated me like a child … now I'll ask questions, because I don't believe that a lot of doctors give you the full picture so now I know to ask questions, and to challenge things.

> (Helen: 18 yrs after diagnosis with Hodgkin's lymphoma)

However, Lesley had not been 'treated like a child' and had been warned that she might face an early menopause, but as she acknowledges, it did not have meaning for her at the time, thus suggesting that even when information is given the implications are not always fully understood.

I didn't think I would have as many sort of ongoing problems, and I find that annoying. You know the menopause thing and … I think they said you may have an early menopause through this, but that didn't mean anything to me really at the time.

> (Lesley: 18 yrs after diagnosis with Hodgkin's lymphoma)

Lesley was 24 when she was diagnosed but still feels that she was unable to take in the implications of the prognosis. If this can be the case at the upper end of the young adult age range, the younger patients may need very careful assessment when they are informed of the late and long-term effects. Louise told me how important it was to have all the information possible to cope with the illness, while she felt that this had been provided in terms of the cancer and her treatment regime during her illness, she too felt unprepared for the longer-term consequences:

I had a letter through my door saying that something to do with your doctor has identified a problem, can you please book a couple of tests. So I phoned up the doctor obviously absolutely distraught … I didn't speak to my doctor, I spoke to an administrator, who said something to me about chronic kidney disease … and it made me even worse … I was so bad that my mum phoned up the doctors, and got angry. So no, I wasn't prepared. I mean I was obviously prepared at the prospect of not being able to be a mum, but anything else then – no.

> (Louise: 8 yrs after diagnosis with Ewing's sarcoma)

Sometimes the lack of information impacts on pragmatic issues such as the need to be re-vaccinated:

I did lack on knowing that I had to get … immunised again. Nobody told me that until 5 years down the line … I didn't actually know I had to do that. Nobody told me so I had to have all my injections again, which was a bit annoying for me. I think the only reason I've mentioned that is because it did actually 'only' take them 5 years to realise 'oh we haven't done this'.

> (Paul B: 11 yrs after diagnosis with non-Hodgkin's lymphoma)

Paul reflected on the potential danger he had been in for the five years during which he was not immunised against any of the diseases that are routinely vaccinated against in childhood. He wondered what the effect on his health would have been and who would have been 'liable' had he contracted, for example, whooping cough. Given the increased susceptibility to infection experienced by some survivors and the threat that infections can a cause, this may be an issue of some significance.

A message to health professionals on preparing survivors was relayed by Debbie as follows:

> I think for health care professionals [to know] ... the most overwhelming thing for me is that those emotions never go away. And so even though it's 20-odd years ago, I can remember most of it as if it was yesterday. And so when you do have to sort of tell somebody, you know things like you've discovered these side effects now and this, that and the other, I think you need to be very, very aware of what it's going to stir up in people ... when I was diagnosed they didn't know any of these side effects. For me personally, I'd always rather know everything. Quite when the right time is to tell somebody that I'm not sure, because you've got so much information to take in at diagnosis. I don't know whether you'd be able to process all of that at the same time. And at the end of the day there is no alternative to having the treatment, because you're going to die ... So obviously to a certain extent the side effects are irrelevant, because if you want to live you've got to do it. So I think ... I mean yes, I think people should know everything.
>
> (Debbie: 22 yrs after diagnosis with Hodgkin's lymphoma)

Ashley, who runs a helpline for people with Cutaneous T-Cell lymphoma (CTCL), has strong opinions on the importance of being informed fully:

> It's a bit like being in an airport and your plane's delayed, and nobody's telling you anything, you could be really badly wound up. But you can wait just as long, if not longer ... if people are keeping you fully informed as to what's going on, you don't worry and you handle it much better ... But some of them [consultants] will try to protect their patients [and think] 'why should I give lots of information out as to what may happen ... with this person's condition when it's entirely possible that it won't progress?'
>
> (Ashley: 37 yrs after diagnosis with CTCL)

We have seen cases where insensitivity or the withholding of information can be detrimental but if a patient is approached with sensitivity and skill, and is prepared for what to expect this can mitigate some of the shock and help establish a willingness to trust that can be carried forward to future encounters with health professionals as well as to prepare for the longer-term consequences. Debbie's experience during her illness was very different from Helen's and shows that the impact of being treated in an age-appropriate fashion can shape perceptions in a lasting way:

> The consultant came round ... he saved me till last, and drew the curtains round the bed and he could see I was upset ... and held my hand and said ... 'look you know, it's got a really, really good prognosis now.' He said, 'we need to find out exactly where it is, but if we've caught it early, and I think we have ... we're looking at [a] 90 per cent survival rate. To be honest Debbie I'd be much, much more upset if I was having to sit here and tell you that you were a diabetic ... because that would never, ever go away. It would have more and more complications, and it would get worse as you get older.' He said, 'This is going to be a real hard slog, and it's not going to be much fun. But you are going to be alright at the end of it.'
>
> (Debbie: 22 yrs after diagnosis with Hodgkin's lymphoma)

Having the contrast drawn between the lymphoma and diabetes appeared to be an enormous psychological boost to Debbie both at the time and as a preparation for her long-term survivorship despite the fact that the consultant appears not to have prepared her specifically for late effects.

Since the time when many of the participants were diagnosed, the advent of the Internet has provided a source of relatively accessible information. However, access to such material without the ability to contextualise the medical detail, coupled with the tendency for worst-case scenarios to be cited, can leave the survivor with unfounded fears. Several of my participants said that a book like the one I was writing (this volume), which was not about the medical issues *per se* but about what it was like to survive and includes accounts from people who have made a success of their survival, was what they would have valued most at the time. As Elaine B said:

> When I was first diagnosed I went to the library and looked in books, and I scared myself to pieces, because all you've got is fatalities ... you can drive yourself more insane by scaring yourself, thinking gosh there's so many died last year, so many ... you know and the prognosis and ... there's not that many survivors, or ... happy stories.
>
> (Elaine B: 15 yrs after diagnosis with Hodgkin's lymphoma)

Picking up on Elaine's comment about the lack of 'happy stories' Richard, as a very long-term survivor, successful professionally and married with a family told me that what he felt young people needed was a role model, or example of a person who had not only survived, but survived well – in short to provide a 'happy story' as an inspiration. To this end he worked for the Teenage Cancer Trust (TCT) to offer hope:

> What I tend to do is to talk about the future and how it's worked for me, so that they can look at me and think 'he's pretty ancient, he's got

married, and he's got a job, and he's got kids, and you know there is a future out there'. And just seeing me walk on stage and be interviewed by other teenagers, you know is ... quite a positive thing to do, as opposed to me try and offer any sort of counselling.

(Richard: 36 yrs after diagnosis with aggressive fibro sarcoma)

It would be tempting to assume that a success story like Richard's would act as a reassurance and inspiration to others, but there is a suggestion from Rowena that other people's recovery is not necessarily a comfort when struggling – as she was – even before she was diagnosed with her second cancer. Rowena said the following about her one visit to a support group:

I actually didn't find that useful at all. I came away probably more depressed than I went, because everyone else was going, 'Oh yes I'm 5 years post-treatment, and I'm fine. And I do this, and I do that.' And I was very poorly at that point. So I didn't find that useful.

(Rowena: 12 yrs after first diagnosis with Hodgkin's lymphoma)

The next chapter picks up in more detail what kind of ongoing support might be found valuable, but it is clear from the contrast between Richard's assumptions and Rowena's experience that the role of 'success stories' is not always interpreted as might be anticipated.

Summary

The long-term and late effects addressed in this chapter are many and varied. They range from visible scarring that causes embarrassment and acts as a constant reminder, to invisible but debilitating exhaustion and lack of stamina. In addition there can be a variety of painful and distressing legacies associated with the illness and its treatment that can last for decades. Despite the range of cancer types experienced and the wide variation in sequelae, a number of issues and themes arose that help us to understand the impact across an extended period of time.

Some of the chapter has focused on a physical legacy that needs medical attention or intervention. However, even survivors for whom the physical consequences were limited were not exempt from worry about how their health might be affected in the long term. It is clear from many of the testimonies that ongoing anxiety about relapse, recurrence or a second cancer permeates survivorship. This effect has been exacerbated by the relatively recent realisation of the late effects of mantle field radiotherapy previously given for Hodgkin's lymphoma. The way in which survivors can best be supported through these concerns is examined in the discussion in the next chapter which is on long-term follow-up.

Health-related anxiety was not limited to the survivors' own health. Several of the participants expressed concerns that their children, or even grandchildren, might have been affected by the cancer, yet according to Levitt and Eshelman (2008) a number of studies have failed to find any increase in the incidence of congenital abnormities or cancers in offspring. Schover suggests that this is a cause for optimism and reiterates the fact that as yet no study has identified excess birth defects after the cancer treatment of one parent, though the genetic damage from cancer treatment may impact rates of early miscarriage or the gender of surviving infants (2007: 256).

However, reassurance based on statistical data from the studies that find no connection with an increase in congenital abnormities or cancers in offspring might be encouraging to survivors. This, though, presupposes that the survivor is willing to articulate their concern to – for example – a GP and that the GP has information on such studies to hand.

The role of the GP is pivotal in the aftermath of the cancer. When follow-up has ended, the GP is often the first port of call if any health concerns arise. For survivors with a legacy of pain access to a pain clinic might be crucial, but there can be difficulty experienced in gaining a referral and an apparent lack of understanding on the part of GPs about the nature of the late and long-term effects and the support that a pain clinic might provide. But survivors also present to their GPs other needs and anxieties. If the GP fails to recognise the role of the cancer history in the survivor's apprehension, if they pathologise anxiety as neurosis or indeed if relatively minor ailments are pathologised as sinister, this can exacerbate what for many survivors is an emotionally loaded medical encounter.

Thus GPs tread a difficult path between taking survivors' concerns seriously while not alarming them unduly and survivors are caught between a need for medical reassurance and a dread of returning to their patient status. So this is a delicate relationship that needs to be handled with care by well-informed health professionals in order for survivors to feel that they are receiving the support they need to manage late and long-term effects and their anxieties about what the future holds.

Not only are a range of late and long-term effects charted here, there are also an equally diverse range of responses to these effects that are not wholly determined by the physical manifestation of the sequelae. Can we ascertain anything about the illness, treatment experience or life context that might shape the way late effects are managed? There are several accounts that suggest that the way the diagnosis is managed at the time can have an ongoing impact on the way in which the illness and survivorship is viewed. Greg's 'glass half full' interpretation seems to be based on an emphasis of his good fortune at having osteosarcoma in his arm and not his leg and Debbie's belief that her cancer diagnosis was preferable to that of diabetes has carried her through survivorship with a positive attitude. Yet those survivors who mistrusted their consultants, who, like Maz, believe they have been misled, kept in ignorance or not treated with sensitivity, carried that mistrust through their survivorship and into future medical encounters.

It was also clear that the information given at the time of diagnosis and treatment needs to be 'age appropriate' thus professionals need to take into account the age and life stage of the young person who may not understand the implications of being told they have a 'malignancy' or a 'lymphoma' and could later be shocked to discover that this means 'cancer'. This too is part of the preparation that survivors need to be able to deal with the late effects and long-term consequences of their illness. However the delivery of 'age-appropriate' information needs to be case sensitive with young people who are at a life stage where they reach levels of understanding and maturity at differing rates. Judgements about competence and capacity must be exercised in order to avoid the danger of the survivor feeling that they have been treated like a child and kept in ignorance or conversely over burdened with information that they cannot process.

Key points

Examples of late and long-term effects

* Physical pain
* Thyroid, digestive and salivary problems
* Scarring
* Permanent change in physical appearance
* General debility and a lowered immunity
* Risk from treatment-related malignancies

Ongoing anxieties

* Fear of future malignancies
* Fear of it being worse a second time round
* Concerns over deteriorating health
* Fear for the health of children and grandchildren
* Possible mistrust of medical professionals
* Fear that GPs may find it hard to keep up with the most recent research on late effects

How to offer the best preparation for survivorship

* A sensitive age-appropriate approach is needed
* Information and honesty are valued
* This can help establish trust for future encounters

---

4 Long-term follow-up and the need for ongoing support

According to Langeveld and Arbuckle (2008), in the past survivors were often left on their own in the post-treatment period but increasing realisation of the complexity of long-term medical and psychosocial sequelae have resulted in late effects clinics being established. These clinics use a multidisciplinary approach to the ongoing support of survivors' needs and clearly play a crucial role in maximising the likelihood of the best outcome for the young person. Recommendations for long-term follow-up include 'yearly physical examination and history, risk modification, avoidance of heavy isometric exercise in higher risk patients, periodic echocardiograms ... and early cardiology referrals for any detected abnormalities.' (Soliman and Agresta 2008: 57)

Different malignancies necessitate differing lengths of time for follow-up. Earle (2007) says that as solid tumours are much less likely to recur after five years surveillance may become less intense over time than, for example, for melanoma which can recur decades later. He documents arguments that surveillance should continue until survival expectation approximates that of matched controls; but for patients with a personal cancer history that puts them at risk of new primaries, Earle suggests life-long follow-up may be appropriate.

According to Jacobs *et al.* (2007) a survey of oncologists suggested that they would value more education and training with respect to the care of long-term survivors. The survey showed that 73 per cent believed they should provide continuing care, 32 per cent reported that they 'always' provided ongoing general medical care including screening, while 47 per cent said that they 'sometimes' provided such services. These results suggest a possible patchiness in provision that can mean survivors may experience different models of support that can vary according to the individual oncologist's approach.

While the importance of such follow-up care is apparent, we need to understand how the provision of this care can be tailored to encourage the optimum use of the service. To do this requires an understanding of the meaning of the experience of attending such a clinic. However, according to Jacobs *et al.* (2007) there have been few studies which have examined the screening behaviours of cancer survivors and this will in turn affect attendance rates and the likelihood of effective monitoring.

The way in which follow-up is regarded can be the cause of some ambivalence; returning to a clinic for follow-up appointments, as Langeveld and Arbuckle (2008) say, can be a stressful reminder. The cessation of active treatment can signify being better, yet 'follow-up' can appear to be contradictory to the notion of recovery. And as Earle (2007) says, the positive benefits of the reassurance, if there has been no recurrence, can be accompanied by inconvenience, stressful testing and awaiting results – all of which can cause anxiety.

Langeveld and Arbuckle (2008) acknowledge that the completion of therapy is a milestone, but one that brings with it the need for a different type of support service. Likewise the completion of long-term follow-up is also a key moment – certainly to be welcomed as it should signify 'cure', but is again a transitional moment after which the discharged patient may still be in need of some form of continued support. Thus this chapter examines – through the testimonies of those who have navigated, and in some cases floundered, through what can be a turbulent and challenging period – not only the experience of follow-up clinics but also what happens after they are no longer offered.

Some of my data collection took place in a long-term follow-up clinic. It was not an age specific clinic; rather it was situated in a general oncology outpatient clinic. This meant that there were people of all ages present, some of whom were in active treatment. A room adjoining the waiting room was used for the administration of chemotherapy and the double doors between the two areas tended to be left open. Patients on chemotherapy drips would wheel their drip stands through the outpatients' waiting area in order to use the bathrooms.

The only patients attending this clinic who fitted my inclusion criteria were young men who had been diagnosed with testicular cancer. It became clear early in my visits to the clinic, that despite having been told that there would be suitable patients for me to interview, the attendance rate was not high and I could never be sure of recruiting any participants. Indeed on one occasion I had expected to be able to interview five patients – yet none of them appeared for their appointments. Of course I can make no assumptions about why that was, neither do I have any details about how far into survivorship they were, nevertheless interviews with some of those who did attend the clinic indicate an ambivalence that may have contributed to the 'no shows'. I have indicated which participants were interviewed in the clinic so that their quotations can be understood in context.

The clinic experience

Ben and Maz whose interviews I quote from later were both patients who did attend their appointments at this clinic and the meaning it had for them gives us some insight into the experience. Despite Ben's expressed need for continuing reassurance and support from professionals, he said the following about the experience of being at the clinic:

> I think the worst thing … one of the worst things is coming here … you know because there's people having chemotherapy, whereas I'm just coming for a bit of a check-up and a blood test you know. And I can't understand why – well I can understand why because it is just simple you know, NHS cost-cutting, you know fit everybody into one clinic – but you could have one doctor on one day do 20 of the people like me for 5 minutes that I go in and see him … and people like me wouldn't have to sit and … you know … I wouldn't say I find it distressing, but I think it's … for the people that are having the chemotherapy I don't think they need an audience … they're getting stressed out because they're having to wait 4 hours for an appointment, which I have done here sometimes. And I just think that could be much better organised … it's more of an inconvenience that's the thing that stresses me out … Right so they're 50 minutes late already and that's normal because this is why I've got … [magazines and stuff] … you know come prepared. It's very normal.
>
> (Ben, in clinic: 4 yrs after diagnosis with testicular cancer)

Ben told me that he did not get paid if he took time off work to come to the clinic; this seemed to be made more complex because of him working night shifts and he had on occasions had to take time off work to attend. He spoke of a friend who faced similar problems:

> Yes, my friend has a big issue with this because … obviously people's sleep patterns are different on nights, because some people like will stay up and then go to sleep, and then get up before they go to work. And some people go to bed as soon as they get home from work. And … the appointments tend be about this time – about eleven o'clock – and I know he's asked for them like early on … but they have [them for] the people that … well to have chemo, which is understandable. But you know for him it's no good at all, because it means he's waiting up until eleven o'clock, he might be here an hour, two hours, then he's got to drive home … obviously you don't want to be using day's holiday for coming here.
>
> (Ben, in clinic: 4 yrs after diagnosis with testicular cancer)

The context of the lives of clinic patients is not something that appears to have been taken into account in the appointments system, if they are paid hourly, work shifts, have transport problems, this can add to the stress of the visit quite apart from any health-related anxiety that might be felt. Ben intimated that the waiting time could be lengthy and this was endorsed by Maz:

> The system here is really slow. If we need to see another … person, like if you need to go from one consultant to another consultant, you're

waiting … and that's what I'm doing all the time … that's the thing, just-waiting for … waiting, waiting, waiting in the hospital – sick of this waiting.

(Maz, in clinic: 4 yrs after diagnosis with Ewing's sarcoma)

The problem of being kept waiting causing additional stress was mentioned by Lisa who told me how much she had dreaded her follow-up appointments that catapulted her back to her treatment phase:

I think you're visiting the past again. You kind of definitely want to try and move on with your life, and this thing's still haunting you. I just remember every appointment my husband came with me, but it was the waiting. You know you had your appointment and it was never at that time. It always seemed it was 3 hours you would be waiting. So that made it even worse. I think if you just went, had the appointment, and came out again, I'd have been fine. But it was the waiting around, which you know it's one of those things on the NHS. You can't criticise but that seemed to make it worse really.

(Lisa: 9 yrs after diagnosis with non-Hodgkin's lymphoma)

Kelly found her dread of follow-up appointments hard to understand as she thought she 'ought' to be simply reassured by them. Nevertheless she also dreaded being 'signed off':

I don't know – I don't why I suddenly start worrying about it around my check-up. Surely I should be more relaxed around my check-up because if there was something they'd find it. But in my mind I start thinking about it a lot more. I think to be told that you're fine, you don't need to come back anymore is probably you know on one hand really exciting, and on the other hand terrifying. So I think to be told that you're all sort of clear and really the hospital doesn't need to see you anymore, but this is here if ever you're worried. Whether it be a phone line that you can call, or a drop in centre. But the phone line would have to be to somebody that you have been involved with.

(Kelly: 7 yrs after diagnosis with non-Hodgkin's lymphoma)

Later in this chapter we examine in more detail what provision might be put in place after follow-up has finished as it is clear that whatever dread the clinic holds, being cut adrift from it is equally alarming. Paul's treatment had finished 9 years previously and his feelings about long-term follow-up seemed to have changed considerably during that period:

It's reassuring now … [but] if I think back I hated coming, and it was kind of like, 'Oh just leave me alone' and my mum … was like, 'No you've got to go'. But I mean to me it was like … it was like something which was like tying me back to this place. So you know when you had to like stay here for a long period of time and I just wanted to leave it. It's like oh no you've got to come back, you've got to think about all that again, you know ... If you're coming back from outside, I mean you're sat with like people who are just going ... still going through that sort of treatment ... and so I guess that ... as an outpatient that jolts you back into where you were at that point, you sit there and kind of think ... and you remember everything ... Yes the smells, some of the smells can just put you right back like ... so ... perhaps having more of a place where there were other people ... who are a similar age.

(Paul, in clinic: 9 yrs after diagnosis with testicular cancer)

Paul B also uses the term 'reassuring' but rather than being 'jolted back' to his treatment phase he worries about what might be found and if a relatively minor ailment might herald a recurrence:

Coming up to your appointment you're obviously thinking well what if they ... if they take your bloods and then you ... they say well ... you have your CT scan results, and mostly at the same time, and you're obviously thinking about what ... what they're going to say. If they have found something and things like that. And then you ... it's strange because you start thinking of all these things that have ... like if you've had a bit of a tickly cough or something, and you mention these things to them, and obviously they think well you've got to have x-rays and things and ... But it's ... at the same time it's reassuring, because when they say well you seem absolutely fine to us, and you know you go, then you're like ... it's like this big sort of come down again then, it's really ... It is reassuring, but at the same time it's quite ... quite scary at the same time.

(Paul B: 11 yrs after diagnosis with non-Hodgkin's lymphoma)

However, despite both the unwelcome anxiety and the welcome reassurance, Paul B had reached the stage after a number of years in follow-up when he sometimes forgot to go. This could illuminate some of the reasons for the poor attendance at the clinic:

I think ... because they do it gradually, you know the time scales of the appointment, I think it does help you in terms of getting away ... from being institutionalised in a way. You're sort of weaning your way off. I mean now ... I even forget about the appointment sometimes, which I shouldn't. And then I suddenly remember I haven't been for a while ... the only time I ... really think about it ... about the illness itself, is when I ... when I have heavy colds and things, because that's obviously the initial symptoms ... and then I suddenly think hang on I haven't been for a while. And then I go find my card that they always give me, which is always at the back of a cupboard somewhere.

(Paul B: 11 yrs after diagnosis with non-Hodgkin's lymphoma)

Paul B's account is similar to many in the previous chapter indicating the underlying concern that relatively trivial symptoms may herald a recurrence, but Paul B's tendency to forget to attend is not the same as Jamie's, he had a record of non attendance at the clinics and he sheds some light on why this was:

> The past year I've got quite ill and I've been moving from place to place as well ... my depression got worse, and for a while I was feeling poorly, so I actually stopped coming to the clinic, because I don't know, it sort of like got into my head to the point where if I go I'm going to get bad news. And I didn't want no more bad news, so I just ... I stopped coming for a bit. But then I thought to myself well it's the last time that I'm coming so I need to go and make sure that it's all clear ... while I've been coming here we're sort of like getting my blood taken, so it was like if anything was actually wrong inside me it'd be picked up straight away, and it would be dealt with. So in a sense it's better to actually come to the clinic, because you know that you're a 100 per cent healthy.
>
> (Jamie, in clinic: 2 yrs after diagnosis with testicular cancer)

So it seems that if feeling dispirited, depressed or emotionally fragile, the fear of bad news can be enough to prevent clinic attendance. Paul indicated that he hated going for follow-up appointments particularly in the early stage. The anticipation of the follow-up appointment was referred to by many participants as causing increasing anxiety in the weeks and days leading up to it. This was replaced by relief when given the 'all clear' and is typified in the following quote from Michael:

> You know when it comes round to my time of the appointment I tend to get a bit ... sort of not anxious, but you know a bit distant maybe for a week or so before, with like work colleagues and friends and things like that. I just try and tuck myself away, knowing that it's coming. Then once it's done, you know back to normal ... if I don't hear anything within a week or a couple of weeks then I assume that everything's okay until the next appointment. So you know it's really sort of from now to over the next week. You know waiting for either the phone call or ... the post dropping through the post box ... from my experience [it's a] top notch, you know grade A service ... Even now people still recognise you when you come in, which for me says a lot that they do actually you know care about what they're doing, and you know they put a lot of time and effort into sort of remembering people's names and they haven't seen me for 6 months.
>
> (Michael, in clinic: 5 yrs after diagnosis with testicular cancer)

Kirsty mirrors Michael's account and her observations bring out the anxiety/relief dichotomy well:

I thought is this normal or is this another symptom of me getting ill again? Things like that would always niggle in the back of my head. So it was kind of like a mixed feeling of anxiety, sort of 'oh do I really want to go and do I want to find out?' But also kind of like 'oh no I'm glad I'm going', because it's almost a relief that you're being seen by sort of someone that I'd actually come to know ... I owed a lot to ... but, yes I mean I always used to get anxious ... it was something that would always remind of what had happened ... But then it was always nice to go back and see [the] doctor ... and always have that reassurance. And you know at the back of my mind I thought well if there is a problem then at least I'm going to sort of you know, be checked over if you know what I mean. But at the same time I always thought 'oh gosh, what if they pick something up' ... there weren't that many symptoms to go with my Hodgkin's lymphoma ... I didn't spot it myself. So there's always that in the back of my head that oh well maybe I haven't spotted something and they'll spot something this time ... then I think oh but then you know in a few years I won't have anything to do with it if you know what I mean. So there's always this almost kind of like ... it is, it's like sort of leaving something behind. And you know not having that reassurance that you're going to go and check, and just like have a once over as it were, and make sure that there's nothing in there ... definitely, I think I will miss it to an extent. But I don't know if that's just because it's kind of like my insurance policy at the moment.

(Kirsty: 5 yrs after diagnosis with Hodgkin's lymphoma)

Greg had had several recurrences of his osteosarcoma and secondaries in his lung. Regarding his attitude to years of follow-up appointments Greg said:

You forget about it entirely, and then suddenly there's a brief build up and, because it's come back several times then there's a day of, you know fear ... you have to look at an x-ray and I remember panicking once and saying 'what's that?' And it's turned out to be my heart or something, and that's fine. But you look at it and you don't know what it's going to be. And you, you're just as used to hearing bad news as good news. But as each year goes by that feeling gets less and less because, because the odds are getting better and better because the first time then you just fear the worst. Second time, gets better, third time. And then by the fourth time, although you can't help but get that fear when you're waiting for the results, it's literally you know for those few hours and the rest of the time it wouldn't occur to me. But you can't actually escape the whole thing until they stop checking you altogether.

(Greg: 19 yrs after diagnosis with osteosarcoma)

Debbie echoed this and said that she had, in the early years of follow-up appointments, been anxious as they approached but that the feelings had eased with time:

> Sometimes I do wonder if for the people having treatment [in the clinic], it's nice for them to see people who are obviously very well coming back. And I mean obviously, in my case, for quite ... even now I'm a lot younger than a lot of the people in the waiting room. And I ... you know I think sometimes it's probably quite nice to see people ... for the people having treatment it's nice to see the survivors, because it ... you know it can be such a slog for you when you're going through it.
>
> (Debbie: 22 yrs after diagnosis with Hodgkin's lymphoma)

It is interesting that Debbie's assumption that patients in treatment would find the presence of long-term survivors reassuring contrasts sharply with Ben's assumption that those undergoing treatment 'do not need an audience'. Debbie told me that she had dreaded being signed off from the clinic as she would have missed the reassurance it gave her – but in the event she was still attending for long-term follow-up when recalled to be screened for the risk of developing breast cancer.

Many of the accounts of follow-up focused on the build up of anxiety, the tedium of waiting and the reluctance to revisit the treatment environment, but Michael's acknowledgement of the welcoming attitude of the staff shows that the negative effects can, for some survivors, be mitigated relatively easily if patients feel that the staff care. But there may be a tension between the bene-fit of returning to where you are known as a patient – and by extension mat-ter personally to staff who had been involved in the treatment phase – and the trauma of returning to the place of treatment as we see from Jack's account:

> I don't like it I must say. I don't like going back to hospital, because you kind of ... I think what it is – I was talking to my friend about this the other day – your body remembers kind of horrors at the speed of which you can handle them. And sometimes, when you go back it's a bit ... it reminds you a bit too much. Because I've actually started to remember more and more the further post treatment I get, about it all ... And in some ways it's a good thing and in some ways it's a bad thing, because the good thing is that it reminds you that you should be grateful for the chance you've been given. Because I go back and I can see obviously patients that are in there at the moment. You know and I see ... I'm very lucky to have you know come out of this ... come out the other side of it. But also it is quite difficult.
>
> (Jack: 9 yrs after diagnosis with Hodgkin's lymphoma)

Jack went on to say that his follow-up did not take place in the same hospital that he had been treated in and if this had been the case he would not have wanted to attend the clinics as the traumatic effect would have been too great. Gillian, 34 years after diagnosis but still in follow-up, similarly said that if the clinic she attended had not been moved to a different hospital she would have been unable to attend. The effect is such that when she returns for follow-up visits she cannot even walk past the hospital where she was treated. So here it seems that as Bob recounted (in Chapter 2) the return to where treatment took place can generate something akin to PTS. This experience is echoed in Helen's account. Helen said that she felt 'brilliant' when the long-term follow-up finished and did not miss the visits in any way despite the subsequent lack of reassurance. It was thus a terrible blow when she found herself back in long-term follow-up for the increased risk of breast cancer but that it was 'a hundred times better' to attend for follow-up at a place where she had not received her treatment:

> They'd said I was in remission for, I think it was 10 years. After that they said basically it's not coming back. But they follow-up because of the age that I was, and I had mantle radiotherapy. So the follow-ups now are, yes in case I get breast cancer ... I've had mammograms probably for the last four years ... Some doctors have been appalling ... I actually asked them to transfer me ... because it really quite traumatised me going which I found particularly traumatic ... I can't go to the consultant's appointment on my own, because I can't sit in that room ... You know they leave you sitting there for ... I mean literally it's usually 5/10 minutes ... you know you're waiting for them to basically tell you you're okay, and everything's clear. So to leave you sitting there ...
> (Helen: 18 yrs after diagnosis with Hodgkin's lymphoma)

If recognition of the emotional cost of attending follow-up is not taken into account the negative impact can be far reaching. As we have seen, visits to long-term follow-up clinics carry with them an emotional significance that cannot be underestimated and when this is not accounted for by staff the impact can be very distressing. For example, I was told by Ruth's mother (see Chapter 2) of an incident that took place at a five year follow-up appointment that demonstrates the importance of getting it right for the patient and their family. On this occasion Ruth was five years out of treatment for ALCL and the appointment was very significant in that it marked the end of the five year protocol she had been treated on. It was also the final appointment with the consultant who had treated Ruth since her diagnosis before she moved onto long-term follow-up with a different consultant. Her mother told me of Ruth's trepidation at revisiting the children's hospital where she had been treated and had undergone so many painful and distressing procedures and where she had come close to death. Ruth had dreaded the appointment and had not wanted to attend. She had reached the stage where she simply wanted to put the experience behind her. However, accompanied by her mother she reported, as requested on the appointment card, to the clinic run by the specialist with whom she had developed a trusting relationship. Once at the clinic the receptionist purported to know nothing of the appointment and said that Ruth's specialist no longer ran this clinic and was not available to be contacted to clarify the situation. Having taken a day (unpaid) from work and having travelled the 150 mile round trip with her mother – herself struggling with ill health – this was a deeply distressing experience. Quite apart from the wasted financial outlay Ruth had 'psyched' herself up for the visit to the hospital and had been dreading it for some time. Ruth and her mother had been contacted by the consultant after their return home and had received a profuse apology. He had in fact been on the premises and told them he should have been paged and would have seen Ruth. However Ruth and her mother had not felt able to insist on this at the time. Ruth and her mother had agreed to make a return visit the following week, but it is possible to envisage a scenario where the young person was unable or unwilling to make the return trip after such an incident.

Ruth's case raises another issue, although 20 at the time of her appointment, the clinic was held in the children's hospital where she had been treated, thus the waiting room was filled with young children. I was told of other long-term follow-up clinics where those treated as teenagers returned to clinics populated predominantly by children as young as 3 years old. Given that follow-up visits could extend in to the patient's 20s, 30s or even older, this can be experienced as additionally distressing and inappropriate.

Jack emphasised that the follow-up clinics should have emotional support as a central component:

> I certainly think follow-up clinics that aren't just to do with the tumour, or the tumour coming back, [what] would be really worthwhile I think [is the] emotional stuff.
>
> (Jack: 9 years after diagnosis with Hodgkin's lymphoma)

In contrast, some of the practical difficulties of attending became clear half way through the interview when Majad suddenly realised that because of the difficulty of finding a parking place he had left his car in a half hour zone and that he would have to go and put more money in the parking meter:

> You know I left my car there, you know half an hour … I couldn't find no parking space and that … I've just seen the time, and I parked it at 20 past and it's bang on 10 to. Normally I used to park it in our street isn't it? But last time when I parked it in our street some smelly guy broke my window … and that's why I don't park it in the streets anymore … Because I don't want anybody breaking my window. I've got a long way me, I live in Lancashire now. So I've got two kids. Last time I left it in Bradford and somebody broke my window. They took my stereo out … and I don't want a ticket as well. I've got too many tickets.
>
> (Majad, in clinic: 7 yrs after diagnosis with testicular cancer)

While the difficulty of parking is a phenomenon familiar to all those who visit a hospital for any reason, when it combines with the profound concern that was clear throughout Majad's interview (see previous chapter) it only served to make him even more anxious. But for Marc who was generally quite laid back about his follow-up care, it was errors on the part of the staff that had caused him most concern:

> I had two minor scares – well it depends how minor ... how you see them. But I had one where they thought I had a lump in my chest and they called me back. It turned out to be a mistake on the film. And another one where they called me back and everybody was clearly flustered about me being there. And then it turned out they'd got the films mixed up, and the person that had the multiple secondary tumours actually wasn't me, and they'd got the x-rays muddled. So they weren't great for me or my family.
>
> (Marc: 21 yrs after diagnosis with osteosarcoma)

The ambivalence was reflected in my interview with Rowena, who indicated that her feelings about attending follow-up clinic appointments would depend on when, in relationship to the appointment, the question was asked:

> If you ask me now I'd say yes I do value it, and it's a relief when I go there. And I know that I'm feeling fine, but when ... it's always as you're coming up to your appointment you always think oh I hope everything's okay. So if you ask me when I ... because I go in October for a check-up. So if you asked me today I'd say yes I really like the follow-ups. When I'm actually going there I think why am I doing this, it's a long way to go just for them to say yes you're fine ... it's a pain having to come once a year, but it is only once a year, and it is a relief when I've been and you've said yes everything's fine.
>
> (Rowena: 12 yrs after first diagnosis with Hodgkin's lymphoma)

At the time of my interview with Louise she attended yearly follow-up clinics and said that she was so much in need of reassurance that she would go more often if she could and wanted the clinics to continue indefinitely. This was partly because her anxiety had been heightened by her aunt's cancer:

> Well my aunt had breast cancer. And she had secondary breast cancer, but it wasn't caught in time. So I'm quite, I guess paranoid about having my check-ups. I'd probably have them every 6 months if they'd let me.
>
> (Louise: 8 yrs after diagnosis with Ewing's sarcoma)

For Richard who attended long-term follow-up clinics for 15 years after his diagnosis with aggressive fibro sarcoma, the visits proved crucial to the early detection and treatment of the testicular cancer he developed some years later. Kate, 31 years after diagnosis was still attending follow-up clinic every 2 years and clearly valued the reassurance they offered. While she said that she did not have a 'pathological dread' of hospitals she told me that she would not want to be visiting the hospital where she had been treated. She also said that the ambience in the waiting room made a huge difference and that even the provision of easy chairs made the experience more acceptable. Reminding us of the accounts in the last chapter is evidence from Kate that even after such a length of time fear of recurrence is ever present:

> I've found [them] quite useful in some ways, simply to go and get the reassurance … for example, I've been having trouble with my neck. I've got arthritis of the spine … I've got discomfort … and because that's the area that I'd had irradiated … I'd been to the doctor, and the doctor had sort of said 'oh there's nothing wrong'. When I went for my next check-up to [the] oncology centre, I was able to say to the specialist there, you know I've been having this discomfort in the neck where I had the radiotherapy. And they sent me for an MRI scan to make sure that there wasn't anything which was in itself quite reassuring, to be able to do that … you worry because however much anybody says 'don't worry', you do worry. [But] the results of my MRI scan got lost between being done and getting to me. And after about 6 weeks of worrying I actually then had to ring up. And this is quite recently. So this is the thing really, this goes back to how it's always there in the background, and you do think that sometimes you know something's going to pop out the woodwork to haunt you from something that's happened so long ago. And I did … I was worried that it might be perhaps a cancer of the thyroid gland, which is a possibility after radiotherapy to the neck. And I suppose that was quite worrying. But it was reassuring then that I was able to have the MRI scan and … which I wouldn't have got from my GP. I think I'd have had to have jumped up and down and banged the table a bit. But they'd sent me, because I'd been … was able to see a specialist. So it's actually quite reassuring to still go.
>
> (Kate: 31 yrs after diagnosis with Hodgkin's lymphoma)

So, if Kate even 31 years after her diagnosis continues to worry and values the opportunity to attend follow-up clinics, what is the impact of their cessation? At one level, the end of follow-up is clearly significant and symbolic of moving on but the ambivalence about attending clinics, the attendant anxiety, the reassurance and the prospect of the loss ongoing support are all encapsulated in Janet's comment:

> It was always a worry. Every time I went it was a worry that they might find something … in some ways whilst it was a worry it was also reassuring. There was that element as well. So in some ways … in actual fact when they did stop the appointments and discharged me … I think it was actually at least 10 [years] I felt quite disappointed when they discharged me in some ways … because even though at that point it had got to a check-up once a year, it was still that contact. It was still knowing that I

was there on the books as it were, and they were still looking out for me. So it was a little bit disappointing really.

(Janet: 27 yrs after diagnosis with Hodgkin's lymphoma)

Janet continued by saying that there was no ongoing support in terms of a self help group or informal way of contacting the clinic and that this had left her feeling unsupported. Elaine B told me that her next appointment might be her last in follow-up and that this would signify the 'next stage of her life'; but clearly her feelings at being signed off were ambivalent:

> I quite like them actually, because at the end of the day they're good for blood tests, and they can feel for lumps and bumps if you're not quite sure. So to me, it's a little bit nerve-racking if you did get a phone call, if there was something untoward with you, but it's quite reassuring to know that you've been for your check-up and you're still okay, because they would get in touch with you otherwise. They've seen me from when I was 23, and now I'm 38. And even if it's just one yearly check-up – they're very you know lovely, friendly people, and 'oh hello Elaine', and all that. So yes, very nice.
>
> (Elaine B: 15 yrs after first diagnosis with Hodgkin's lymphoma)

So Elaine B, like Michael, valued the personal touch of being remembered and having her first name used, for her the return to the hospital where she had been treated was reassuring. While not all participants felt as positive about the follow-up clinics and the way they were managed, most would at some stage face the termination of this source of monitoring and several indicated that this would leave them feeling unsupported and insecure. This raises the question of what kind of ongoing support can be offered to those not still attending clinics or for those who find the clinic visits traumatic and would not want to continue in the longer term. It is to this need for some continuity of assurance that we now turn.

The need for ongoing support

There are a number of indications in the earlier accounts that the termination of long-term follow-up care is both welcomed and dreaded. It might be, as Elaine B indicates, that it signifies the next stage of life and thus must be embraced as symbolic of progress and confirmation of cure and survivorship. Alternatively – or even concurrently – it can leave the patient feeling unsupported and insecure without the regular reassurance offered at the clinics even when those clinic visits have caused anxiety and emotional distress. As Julie said:

> When it got to 10 years, they sort of said, 'oh we don't need to see you anymore' ... that was really hard to let go from the monitoring ... I don't

know if I'm quite ready for that ... he is keeping me on for a bit because I've actually got to go for a bone scan later this week, so just precaution- ary thing or whatever. But as soon as that's done he's going to discharge me – I hate that word, because that puts the fear of God into me. Discharge me! Then there's nobody to ask or you know, if I've got a niggle ... you know what I mean?

(Julie: 15 yrs after first diagnosis with Hodgkin's lymphoma)

The combination of being cast adrift from support coupled with the tendency to have ongoing concerns about health (as discussed in Chapter 3) raises the issue of what provision might be made for something less formal than clinical follow-up, that could be accessible, as and when discharged patients feel the need for support or reassurance, or if they simply have the need to talk. Jack envisaged a variety of needs:

Knowing there's a support group there for you I suppose, it would be ... it would be a big thing ... just knowing there's a ... you had a consultant there who was ... who knew people who could physically, or who knew people you could go to about certain things. Maybe an annual coun- selling session as well or ... just someone to talk things through with, because sometimes there are things that you don't want to talk to your friends about. I mean telling your friend that you can't have kids is just not something you [do].

(Jack: 9 yrs after diagnosis with Hodgkin's lymphoma)

Dan had been offered what he called a 'lifetime membership' of the follow-up clinic to which he could return at any time. He was one of the people who valued the return to a place where he was known and thus welcomed this direct route to support should he require it:

At the moment I almost quite revel in the fact that I ... you know I'm fine, if I'm not fine then I'll be told ... I did actually get quite a lot of reassur- ance when I went last time and they said that that the clinic is a sort of open clinic if you ever have any worries or concerns you don't need to go through the GP and through the system again – I can just go straight into the clinic and they'll check it out ... and that's sort of a lifetime member- ship ... I do get a lot of reassurance from that because ... I mean I know I was going on about saying how I'm not worried, but obviously it's defi- nitely nice to be looked after from that point of view ... I think being able to have a hotline to the clinic is very nice, very nice indeed ... the nurses in the clinic seem to have always been there and will always be there sort of thing. And every time I go in they're absolutely lovely, they know exactly who I am ... and so that's brilliant ... there's something really lovely about that because you feel just secure I suppose and that some- body knows your history and will know if anything's not right; it's a really brilliant thing to have ... I think probably what I've got is one of the best things that can be provided long term, and that's being able to just go in if I need to, if I have a concern. And I suppose maybe a phone number you could ring for that would be a good thing if you had any concerns ... quite genuinely I am really pleased about that because I know they've got all my records there. And that's for life you know ... I think that's the best thing to be honest, because other than that I think it's important to move on. And I wouldn't particularly want to be in a support group now. I mean okay I'd be able to help other people, but ... apart from feeling good about myself, I don't think I would get anything from it personally ... I think there comes a point when ... particularly with cancer, where you really need to get on with life ... I've never actually been a part of a support group – although it was offered to me – and partly that was because I already had good support from my family.

(Dan: 5 yrs after diagnosis with testicular cancer)

It seems significant that despite the obvious value Dan placed on the offer of continuing support from people he trusted and valued who could reassure him from a medical perspective, he felt that the time had come for him to move with his life. The implication here seems to be that a support group would not represent 'progress'. Perhaps he feared the identity of being a survivor would become too significant at a time when he should be moving on, as Elaine B said, to the next stage of life. It may also be significant that Dan further observed the tendency for men to not go to the doctor so there may be a gender difference to be taken into account in the appropriate provision of ongoing support. In contrast Paul expressed a need for some ongoing support system that might entail belonging to a group despite the fact his initial reaction would have been to refuse:

I read a book ... and actually I didn't plan it, I was in a bookshop and I just saw this book. It's by this lady who had breast cancer actually ... and I read that and I was like, 'Oh yes, yes that's exactly ... ' you know. And there was some bits – not everything because I mean she had a family – I read it and thought yes that was ... If we could have had some access to some place where other people can talk ... I didn't expect it, but when he said that sort of like you've got one more year [at the follow-up clinic] and then we'll let you go, I suddenly felt what if something happens the year after that? What will I do then? ... if there had of been some sort of group ... I think if somebody had suggested it I probably would have said 'no', but then I would have thought about it and thought 'yes'.

(Paul, in clinic: 9 yrs after diagnosis with testicular cancer)

Kelly suggested a slightly different model than a normal support group, and it seems particularly significant that she mentions the importance of it being 'age appropriate':

I've always kind of liked the idea of ... not so much a support group, but kind of being able to ... go out socially with some of the people ... that have been treated around the same time as you. Some kind of group, which would obviously get bigger as other people joined it, but just something that you could opt in or opt out of. And just some kind of outlet with other patients ... it could be age appropriate as well.

(Kelly: 7 yrs after diagnosis with non-Hodgkin's lymphoma)

Kirtsy was concerned that after follow-up had finished she would be without support and knew that to share her anxiety with her mother would place too big a burden on her, thus some form of after care support was necessary:

I mean my mum especially, as any parent would be, if I ever said oh I'm a bit worried about something like this, I mean I know she'd panic ... So even if there was just someone to talk to ... you know that external outlet that I can you know, use to sort of voice what's on my mind. Whether it's you know relevant or not. So maybe something like that's kind of completely separate to anything you know at home or your friends and family, and things like that ... just someone to talk to that can reassure you, or sort of give you advice would be good because you know it's kind of like 'oh is this worth bothering someone about, or am I just being paranoid?'

(Kirsty: 5 yrs after diagnosis with Hodgkin's lymphoma)

Julie had no ongoing advice and support after her diagnosis with Hodgkin's lymphoma and spoke of the key role played by the Lymphoma Association that provided both information and a network that lessened isolation. Julie emphasised the importance of the support group without which she would have been left in ignorance about many aspects of her illness:

It was about 1992, so we're talking about 15 years. And it's amazing how much things have changed in that time, because obviously I didn't have a computer, I didn't have the Internet ... I didn't know any young person who had had cancer. I didn't know any information about the disease itself, and the prognosis and the ... basically what it is and you know, what the theories are about it. And so I knew nothing, absolutely nothing. And it was because, you know, I went to the support group. It was just a helpline then and a few sort of fact sheets.

(Julie: 15 yrs after first diagnosis with Hodgkin's lymphoma)

However, support groups are not for everyone and, as evidenced in many observations earlier, it seems that Lisa's reluctance to attend was at least in part because they were held in the hospital where she had been treated – even catching sight of her oncology consultant when she was a maternity patient caused her distress:

I did go to some support groups ... at the very beginning when I was in remission ... I did go, but I didn't get a great deal of benefit from it ... some of the support groups we went to were back at the hospital. Well that was the worst thing for me. You're going back to the floor that you were on when you were really poorly, and it's just revisiting those dark days when you don't really want to go back to the hospital. Perhaps ... it was actually in the wrong place ... My consultant – not a very good bedside manner – totally freaked me out ... I absolutely was terrified by her presence ... I had my children in the same hospital. And I think we managed to see her at some point. And I just saw her from a distance and I froze with horror, seeing her ... It just reminded me of the bad times. I don't want anything to do with her. And even though I ... really respect her as a professional ... she obviously treated me very well. And I have no concerns about how she treated me. But I can't stand the sight of her if you see what I mean.

(Lisa: 9 yrs after diagnosis with non-Hodgkin's lymphoma)

However, despite Lisa's reluctance to revisit her place of treatment or belong to a group or, she would consider supporting others:

I'm the type of person that doesn't really want to talk to other people about it. And that's how I seem to cope with it. I didn't want to compare stories with anyone else on what their treatment ... because I think if something bad had happened to someone then that would have, I think destroyed me really. But now I wouldn't mind being a buddy ... to someone. I think because I'm so many years down the line ... I could perhaps do that now.

(Lisa: 9 yrs after diagnosis with non-Hodgkin's lymphoma)

In the absence of any ongoing support or 'buddying' Elaine looked at the Lymphoma Association website in order to generate some connectedness with others who had undergone the same experience:

I don't know, I mean I sort of ... sort of probably sounds awful, but I sort of have a look at the ... sort of the message board and just you know, I ... because it's sort of other people and their stories, and I just sort of want to know what other people deal with it, or what they've had. But I mean I find that quite hard in some ways, because you know I do feel like I've come through it very lightly. So I feel like almost a bit of a fraud you know, having a look and ... you know other people's experiences, because most of the other people you read about are sort of so much worse affected by it.

(Elaine: 5 yrs after diagnosis with Hodgkin's lymphoma)

Gillian emphasised that while information was crucial it needed to come from a trusted source and be put into context otherwise – as she found – it was alarming and often offered only the worst-case scenario:

> Information is useful … but the right sort of information. And I do think with computers now it can be quite dangerous, because it's easy to get onto sites that could frighten. Some of the American sites … can be quite frightening. [I had] no one to turn to. I only had my nursing textbooks and they all said I wasn't going to survive. Literally, I mean … according to them I wasn't going to survive, but you know that is all I had. There needs to be … somebody to talk to … there's no point having this information, and … getting completely frightened. There's got to be a contact, an actual person that you can contact. You know maybe say you know, you've read this, and then put it into context. It's so easy to take information out of context.
>
> (Gillian: 34 yrs after diagnosis with Hodgkin's lymphoma)

Although this volume does not offer any medical information or advice, in relationship to my study Gillian said: 'I mean I do feel that what you're doing is great … it can help other people to know you're not isolated'. However, Jamie thought a support group might be valuable not only for information and reassurance, but also for him to be able to reinforce his sense of survivorship in that he could reassure others 'worse off' than him. Unlike Elaine who felt a 'fraud' when faced with others who had had worse experiences, in some sense Jamie felt that this would help his self esteem:

> I suppose in a sense a support group, because a support group for … would actually help my self esteem as well because there'd be people that were worse off than me in there, so in a sense I could sort of like reassure them. And there'd be people that were in the same boat as me that it's affected them more, so again I could sort of like say to them well you'll be alright, I've been there, I've done that, and I'm fine through it. So a support group really and truthfully would be a good thing …
>
> (Jamie: 2 yrs after diagnosis with testicular cancer)

But while a support group may provide emotional support what it cannot do is offer a medical interpretation of worrying symptoms. As we saw in Chapter 3, many survivors have ongoing anxieties about their health and to have the opportunity to have concerns allayed or to be referred quickly for investigation is of central importance. Julie, unlike Dan, had sought the advice of her GP but her quest for reassurance was not satisfactory, the result being that she would be reluctant to seek another appointment:

> Once I went to my GP when my glands were you know really swollen under my neck, and I was just thinking … I was a bit worried. And I found him to be sort of really quite sort of patronising that you know, it

was just glands having come up. And I thought well, you know he could have been a little bit more sympathetic ... I just wanted somebody to sort of you know say it is ... I just needed sort of well you know, that 'yes it's absolutely fine ... I'll have a quick prod and sort of see what's what'. But I just felt him to be you know really quite patronising ... it was just, you know the way he said it. And I just thought well ... he could have been you know, more sympathetic to what I was going through, because you know part of it is, you know in my head. And I just need that reassurance. And I sort of thought then you know, if I had any concerns I wouldn't necessarily want to go back to my GP. But then on the other hand sort of actually phoning up the hospital and saying I need to make an appointment myself seems like such a huge thing, because it really would be saying that there is something there.

(Elaine: 5 yrs after diagnosis with Hodgkin's lymphoma)

So for some there seems to be a 'gap' in provision between the GP and the hospital and this feeling is endorsed by Kate. There was a strong intimation from her that the experience of consulting a GP might be problematic so to simply be redirected by a helpline to a General Practice would not necessarily be very helpful:

I think it's quite counter productive when a helpline says well you ought to go and see your doctor, because that might be the truth, but actually most people have rung a helpline because they don't sort of ... they can't ... you know either can't see the doctor, or they don't get on with them, or they don't think they're going to get a good service. So they want something a bit more specialised than the GP's own knowledge.

(Kate: 31 yrs after diagnosis with Hodgkin's lymphoma)

Possibly the need for support is shaped to some extent by the informal support network available to survivors:

I mean I never used the sort of user groups or anything like that at the time, because I'd got people close to me that I could talk to anyway. But I could completely understand that it would be different, you know if people are on their own or don't have that kind of support, then yes, it would be vital that that was there I'm sure ... [but] I wouldn't go on a website.

(Lesley: 18 yrs after diagnosis with Hodgkin's lymphoma)

However, while informal support might be of emotional benefit, it would still not meet the need for easily accessible and sympathetic medical advice. While some people might find an online information or support network beneficial not everyone would use this medium with ease. Paul too said a website would not appeal to him after the eventual finish of his follow-up clinic appointments:

> If I did think there was something wrong, like if glands came up or any-thing like that, and I thought hang on there's one or two symptoms that are ... I'd probably just go through the normal channels – go to the GP and then get referred, and so on and so forth. But I think because I've got, again the family there, I don't really need to reach out to the other people.
>
> (Paul B: 11 yrs after diagnosis with non-Hodgkin's lymphoma)

So as with Lesley the support of family appears to have been crucial and it also seems that Paul's GP was more sympathetic to his concerns than was Elaine's. Kate pointed out that some of the big cancer charities were largely engaged in fundraising for research rather than offering support to individual patients, but she used her experience of another patient support group that she sug-gested as a possible model:

> A while back I went to a meeting of a group for people with ME ... about eight or ten of them who met for lunch in a pub, and talked about having ME. And they weren't fundraising; they were just meeting to share an experience. And just to meet somebody who's got the same thing that they have, so they don't think they're going mad ... It was small, it was local ... I think they had one person who was sort of nominally in charge, but I think all she did was say yes we'll be back here, you know third Thursday next month kind of thing ... they were just getting together ... and that might be a good model for a very small informal group, to get together just to meet other to make you feel better.
>
> (Kate: 31 yrs after diagnosis with Hodgkin's lymphoma)

The importance of a support group was emphasised by Mary, who unlike most other participants had become firm and lasting friends with a fellow patient:

> I joined a cancer support group. The first sort of three episodes of Hodgkin's, I was very much head in the sand like, 'I'm not ill, I don't want anything to do with cancer. I don't want to meet any other patients.' I didn't have the opportunity to meet any anyway. But the last lot the con-sultant there was very keen to set up a support group. And I was in that first batch of people ... Oh it was fantastic. And also of course I met the first few other people with Hodgkin's ... That's where I met Liz. Liz and I have been firm friends ever since ... So that has been an absolutely fun-damental you know friendship. But also in the support group it was a mixed support group. So of course our prognosis was quite good being Hodgkin's patients. But a lot of other people in that group died ... We

actually went to 11 funerals ... in 2 years, in our early 20s, where we lost friends of ours who were maybe not that much older than us, because they were sort of maybe in their 30s or 40s. Most of them, in fact, breast cancer patients. And we used to go to these funerals together. But it was ... I often look back and think 'God that was such an unusual experience'. At the time it felt normal because that's what we were doing. But actually I look back and now realise that was a totally abnormal experience for a 21/22 year old ... I would certainly not wind the clock back and not do it. But I think it certainly changed my view of things. It made me meet lots of people I wouldn't have otherwise have met.

(Mary: 24 yrs after diagnosis with Hodgkin's lymphoma)

It is clearly not possible to attend as many funerals and lose as many friends as Mary and not to be permanently affected by the experience. As she says it is a 'totally abnormal' experience to have in early adulthood and is bound – as she acknowledges – to change attitudes and the approach to life. However, it would be less likely to lose members of a long-term survivors' group than of a support group of newly diagnosed or discharged patients. Michael said that as a long-term survivor himself he, like Jamie, would now get a great deal out of helping someone going through the experience whether through a group or individually as he realised how important it is to have a role model of someone who has survived long-term and been successful.

I would certainly offer any help to anybody, you know albeit I'm not a professional ... but you know, just be there, and provide support. I think a massive thing that helped me at the time was reading Lance Armstrong's book actually ... a friend of a friend sort of found out that obviously I'd got the cancer, and lent me the book. And I just ... I could completely relate to everything that he'd been through. And it was just like seeing it written down and thinking you know, I'm not actually the only person in the world. And look at him, what he's turned out to be. And because of that you know, I'm back into sports, I'm playing more sports than ever. And you know, just living everyday as it is really.

(Michael: 5 yrs after diagnosis with testicular cancer)

Michael is not the only survivor to have mentioned the importance of a published personal testimony. The assurance, not only of life after cancer but successful, productive life, coupled with the knowledge that the experience has not only been shared by others but others who can act as an inspiration, seems to be of great meaning and significance.

Understanding the issues facing patients at the end of long-term follow-up, John, in his role as a cancer nurse had undertaken a study of their needs:

I did an audit ... looking at long-term survivors patients' views on discharge. And clearly some patients are happy to be discharged while others just want that safety mechanism, knowing that there is somebody at the hospital ... those patients that want to be followed up long-term do very much value the clinics. And they sometimes can't understand, you know when you try to explain to them that there's not a great deal of value in a once yearly appointment. And I think, with the greatest respect to GPs, many patients are a little bit fearful of being referred for their annual check-up to the GP ... not the one with the expertise in you know, any particular cancer.

(John: 33 yrs after diagnosis with Hodgkin's lymphoma)

The majority of the reflections on ongoing support needs were contributed by those not currently in follow-up. This suggests that while the need continues it may not be anticipated until the follow-up clinics – viewed with ambivalence by many – are terminated. It is at this point that feelings of insecurity manifest in anxiety and isolation and there is recognition that some form of back up is needed.

Summary

While shared concerns are addressed by the participants in this chapter it is also apparent that one model or solution to follow-up and ongoing support would not be applicable to all survivors – there are a variety of needs expressed thus indicating that a range or flexibility in services may be needed. This may also change as the length of survivorship alters the quality of the experience and the requirements that accompany it. In the same way that transition from childhood to adulthood is not a fluid process and there is vacillation in relationship to need, dependency and independence, the same processes are affecting the separation from dependence on follow-up clinics. The ambivalence that such dependence engenders is clear, nevertheless, there is an expressed need for continuing support and reassurance, to be picked up and laid aside as necessary. There is enough evidence in the accounts of what is found helpful – and unhelpful, and what might be acceptable in terms of ongoing support, to make some observations on how to maximise the chance of offering appropriate provision.

It is clear that some survivors value the support at a clinic where the staff are familiar with them and their histories are understood, while it is equally clear that the return to the place of treatment can trigger something akin to PTS for others. How can such a dichotomous response be understood and managed? It may be that experiences during the treatment period and feelings about the engagement of staff and the personal interest expressed in their individual circumstances shape the way future contact is viewed. It was those care environments where people felt valued – as opposed to those where the treatment might have been excellent but the personal interaction had been brusque – that could be revisited with equanimity. Thus it is important that professionals know that attitudes to follow-up can be primed during treatment and may continue to shape medical encounters for many years.

Several participants indicated that a separate clinic for long-term follow-up, that may also be age specific, would make the ordeal much less onerous than sitting in a general oncology outpatients clinic with patients (mostly much older) who are currently in treatment. There were also features of the clinic that might be considered trivial – particularly in relationship to the potentially life changing or even life-threatening news that might be heard at a follow-up clinic – that could transform the experience. The physical comfort of the waiting area, the provision of easy chairs, the minimisation of the waiting time, the convenience of the appointments offered and the friendliness of the reception staff can all make a profound difference when under stress. Of course such considerations could be applied to any hospital clinic appointment, but what is different with long-term follow-up is precisely that it is 'long term'. If commitment is to be sustained across many years – in some cases for life – the prospect of visits stretching into the future has to be sustainable emotionally as well as practically. The emotional component of both attendance and the impact on the survivors' lives also needs to be embedded into the consultation alongside the medical aspects.

In the same way that the follow-up clinic appointments could be viewed as both anxiety provoking and reassuring, so too can their termination. Clearly whatever the experience of follow-up – positive or negative – the cessation of the long term monitoring carries with it a profound symbolic meaning. It can act as a signifier of cure and recovery while at the same time leaving the survivor feeling cut adrift and isolated. Most of the accounts suggest that something is necessary to fill the void, even if it remains unused, the knowledge that there is an option to access expert support or advice easily or even informally, is significant. So, what might support look like?

Not only are clinic appointments viewed with contrasting perspectives, so is the need and preference for how ongoing support might be provided. It is clear that support groups are not for everyone, though even those that did not feel they would use them might contribute to the support of other patients earlier in their journey. The 'lifetime membership' model may be one option that would allow the referral route through a GP to be circumvented and direct and easy access to a clinic to be arranged. GPs were viewed with ambivalence and while some participants felt supported, it was clear that others did not want to have to be channelled through a preliminary appointment in order to be seen by a specialist. Even a helpline to act as a filtering system so that possibly unnecessary anxieties could be allayed, or a rapid and easily organised clinic appointment could be made, would be welcomed. This might help to allay some of the concerns raised by accessing information via the Internet that is seen out of context, with no guarantee of its quality and with no ability to discuss its significance with an expert.

However, information provided in a more contextualised form from, for example, the Lymphoma Association, was regarded highly. Such an illness specific site was seen to address survivors directly, be trustworthy, authoritative and up to date with the most recent developments in treatments. The extension of such online support might therefore act as an intermediary between the unmediated, unregulated and occasionally alarmist data on the Internet, and making an appointment with the GP or accessing another source of medical advice such as a helpline.

Readers may ask what the earlier accounts have to say about the age at which the cancer was diagnosed and treated. Many of the issues, problems and challenges experienced by the participants might apply to survivors of cancers diagnosed at any age – so can life stage as a distinct and defining feature be applied to the follow-up experience? I suggest that while reactions to many of the frustrations, anxieties and difficulties might be universal there are some aspects of the experience that relate to age and life stage. First, the prospect of long-term follow-up is likely to occur at a moment in time when the young people have already had their life trajectories altered abruptly and their plans thrown into turmoil, thus the prospect of future visits extending for years into the future may appear very dispiriting – they are better but they are still 'patients'. It is also the case that attendance may be affected, as we saw in the case of the young men with testicular cancer who did not appear for their appointments. Sustaining commitment to attending clinics – particularly when career, education or other life plans necessitate moving away from the area – may prove disruptive to adolescent and young adult life. In contrast, survivors of childhood cancer and older survivors may have more settled lives where geographic mobility and lifestyle are not such an issue.

Thus, without in any sense wishing to diminish the experience of follow-up in other age groups, it seems from the testimonies of my participants that for follow-up to be of optimum benefit and to cause minimum anxiety, some life stage issues may need to be built into the design for provision.

Key points

* Long-term follow-up clinics can offer much needed reassurance
* However, clinic staff at every level need to take account of the emotional cost of attendance
* Non attendance may denote emotional or psychological problems
* The cessation of long-term follow-up may be welcomed but can result in considerable insecurity
* The option of some form of ongoing support would be welcomed by most long-term survivors
* Such support needs to be offered in a variety of forms such as: support groups; drop in clinics; telephone helplines; trustworthy illness specific websites and direct access to medical information
* The opportunity to help others through the experience and to act as mentors may be welcomed

5 The emotional legacy
How it changes philosophy and perspective

As we saw in the previous chapter, there is a powerful emotional and psychological aspect to survivorship which manifests itself not only in relation to attendance at clinics and the post traumatic effect that this may have on some survivors, but it also permeates aspects of daily life in ways which may be unexpected. McQuellon and Danhauer (2007) suggest that 30 per cent to 50 per cent of cancer survivors may experience distress significant enough to warrant professional intervention at some time during their survivorship. These authors also state that some survivors say they feel they will never 'return to normal' even after a declaration of survival because they carry a constant sense of foreboding and worry – as seen in the previous chapter – about recurrence.

Soliman and Agresta (2008) report studies that have shown an increase in depression that can be attributed to chronic physical sequelae and that the emotional damage can manifest as PTSD. Similarly, Nezu and Nezu (2007) argue that as cancer engenders many stressors this can lead to a significantly compromised quality of life affecting many areas – even for those people who had previously coped well with major negative life events. If this can be the case for older survivors whose life experience may have helped them develop coping skills, how much more problematic might the emotional impact be for survivors of adolescent young adult cancer?

Langeveld and Arbuckle say that while the post-treatment phase may come with the promise of happiness, once the survivor has been given the 'all clear' this can in reality be a very emotionally draining time (2008: 149). Feelings of relief may be accompanied by guilt, anger, anxiety, blame, loss and fear; some of which we have already seen manifested in the previous chapters.

However, in spite of the suggestions earlier that all indicate a negative effect, McQuellon and Danhauer (2007) argue that some survivors may actually find some benefits, have improved psychosocial functioning and a greater appreciation of life. The section at the end of this chapter consists of extracts from my participants' interviews that indicate this can indeed be the case. Thus the negative expressions of emotional dysfunction or distress should be understood in conjunction with the positive accounts included later in the chapter.

However, whether negative or positive, there is likely to be some emotional effect and Kelly acknowledges that while there is evidence of the emotional needs of adolescents and young adults with cancer 'our understanding needs to be developed further' (2008: 33). I would argue that if the state of knowledge surrounding the emotional needs and impact during the illness is limited, our knowledge about how the emotional impact plays out throughout the remainder of life is even more limited.

To some extent an 'emotional' element is integral to the accounts throughout this volume and in separating material for this chapter it has been difficult to know where to draw the boundaries. However, this chapter takes as its focus not only the emotional effects, but also the way in which the illness has shaped how life is approached, how risks are perceived, and asks if a fundamental change of philosophy is central to the experience of survivorship.

The emotional impact

Julie identified one emotional impact of the illness being a tendency to worry about her children's health and well-being. To some extent this may have been because all three of her surviving children were on the autistic spectrum and one child had died at birth:

> I do definitely [worry] with my children ... I definitely do ... all three of my children are on the autistic spectrum, which is really unusual. And they've had really kind of odd illnesses ... And the number of times I've had said to me, things like, 'The chances of that happening are very low. You needn't worry about that.' And then it happens. And I feel like well, I tend to think of myself as always being in that percentage of people that it happens to. And I'm okay about that, because that's ... I'm sort of like well yes, that's fair enough, but let's just recognise that and get on with it. Recognise it and do something about it. But I always feel like I'm in a fight ... I think people tend to think I overreact a lot about things ... my youngest son, Will, has a problem with allergies and asthma and things like that. And I wanted him to go and see an immunologist in Manchester, which I didn't think was an unreasonable request. But the local paediatrician wasn't keen, didn't feel it was necessary. And I just felt he needed a second opinion.
>
> And when ... anyway eventually this referral went through, and I actually got to see the letter, because it was in my son's notes. And it was the most derogatory, putting-down letter, about me, you could imagine, saying that I take things way out of proportion. And it was a real shock. And just seeing how people must view me, you know some people anyway. And it does make you question, I think well do I take things way out of proportion? And you know, and overreact. I don't know, I question myself about it now. But I am very, very cautious,

I'm a very cautious person. That's me, I'm very, very cautious about things.

(Julie: 15 yrs after first diagnosis with Hodgkin's lymphoma)

It seems that Julie has braced herself to expect the worst because that is what her experience suggests can happen despite reassurances on the odds. Her cancer has coloured her perception of herself and the people she loves as 'unlucky' – always in the minority of those whom, whatever the odds against it, disaster will strike. But in addition to her understandable fear of the worst it seems that she has been constructed by others as unreasonably anxious in their apparent failure to comprehend the impact of her own illness on her management of her sons' health problems. Similarly, for Kirsty, the fact that the unthinkable had happened, seemed to have left her with the fear that anything could happen and that she had no control over life events, yet this was accompanied by an almost contradictory 'if it happens, it happens' attitude:

I think a big part of it is the kind of lack of control over everything that happens in my life ... because that happened to me, I thought oh God, well anything can happen now. There's nothing I can do ... I went to Spain with my mum for my birthday, and I was absolutely terrified of getting on a plane. And I'd never, ever, ever been terrified of flying. And it was just things like that. And I just thought 'oh God, oh you know why is this?' And obviously I went into sort of like a little self analysis, and thought well maybe it is because I'm scared that something can happen now, because I'm worried that things are out of my control ... but then I guess it's kind of swings and roundabouts, because at the same time I think well you know, if it happens, it happens, because I think there is kind of the happy-go-lucky attitude that I think anyone would sort of like you know take on after something like that. But it is weird ... my fear of risk is something I can't control, and maybe perhaps my sort of like well what the hell attitude, or something like that. I don't know whether ... like because certainly I think it's probably made me think well you know life's too short.

(Kirsty: 5 yrs after diagnosis with Hodgkin's lymphoma)

Like Kirsty, in the following account the combination of a tendency to worry coupled with a sense of perspective conferred by the illness is articulated well by Kelly:

I'm a worrier ... but I think it's just given me perspective. So I'll worry about something, and then every so often I'll just stop and I'll just think there really is no point in worrying about this. It's not going to get you anywhere; you're making yourself unhappy, just stop. And that's because of what I've been through ... I sort of think it's because I look back on what I've been through and think well actually I have got that inner strength. But I know that I can get through this. And I'm going to get through whatever this little minor stress is too, so I can just stop and not worry about it so much.

(Kelly: 7 yrs after diagnosis with non-Hodgkin's lymphoma)

The issue of 'risk-taking' and 'caution' raised by both Julie and Kirsty is picked up again later in this chapter. However, Debbie whose earlier treatment for Hodgkin's lymphoma had left her at risk of breast cancer talked about the emotional impact when she first found out about the risk. She was catapulted back into an emotional turmoil that she had previously been able to leave behind her:

And it brought back an awful lot of feelings … it stirred up an awful lot of emotions about the time. And I think … I think the vulnerability that it brought back. And now [with] my own children, and it was that sort of feeling of I've got to get them a bit older before anything can happen to me. And you know that sort of thing. And I found it very, very unsettling for a couple of weeks. And, you know it's all fallen back into place now. But I was surprised at the strength of emotion after all this time … I think some of my emotions are tied up with having had my husband walk out on me when the children were little, with a nervous breakdown, and having to have brought them up on my own, and turned everything round and I've started teaching since then, which I never thought I'd do. And I'm not quite sure where the lymphoma emotions stop and the sort of surviving the end of the marriage emotions kick in. I suspect these days they're all very tied up together probably.

(Debbie: 22 yrs after diagnosis with Hodgkin's lymphoma)

Julie and Debbie have both experienced difficulties that it could be argued have no connection with their cancers yet separating the emotional impact of those events from the emotional legacy of the cancer is problematic, it seems that there remains an underlying emotional vulnerability that is not far beneath the surface and easily resurrected. Ashley describes it as being akin to PTS:

It's a little bit like Post Traumatic Stress (PTS) syndrome associated with being held hostage or being in an accident that you've survived and come away from … I've read a lot about people who've been in a situation where they have no control of danger to their lives. And you could argue that having this kind of diagnosis is the same sort of thing … The trauma associated with being in a hostage situation, for example, is well understood these days. A lot of studies have been written as to the syndrome itself, and how when you have no control over that situation and somebody else has got control, like the disease has got control over you, that has a fundamental effect on the whole of your being … But that changes, that evolves ... over the years to varying degrees depending on how the prognosis has changed ... with a lot of people who don't have [the] 100 per cent all clear, who are told you know that they need to come back for tests ... there's still the threat. This Damoclean sword that's hanging over them that will colour their lives if they let it. And that's the key – if they let it.

(Ashley: 37 yrs after diagnosis with CTCL)

Ashley infers an element of choice over the matter with his 'if they let it' comment, yet it is interesting that Helen uses the word 'obviously' to explain her depression as if there were in effect no choice:

I obviously got very depressed, and quite suicidal. And afterwards I went to university and I thought I was a couple of times having panic attacks. But from what I understand now they were just very serious anxiety attacks, because I understand a bit more about it now I've seen the psychologist ... I don't really trust people that much ... I'm not great trusting sort of new people if you see what I mean ... because a lot of people at the time didn't know how to deal with my illness, which is fair enough when you're 17. But they didn't really know how to deal with it. And people let you down, you know ... When I was talking to the psychologist, that's part of the problem that causes my anxiety is that I don't want to be different, I want to be like everybody else ... So, that I guess has now caused, as an adult ... well it's a cumulative effect.

(Helen: 18 yrs after diagnosis with Hodgkin's lymphoma)

Helen's observation on her age at the time of treatment resulting in people not knowing how to deal with her coupled with her 'which is fair enough' perhaps indicates she feels unconscious self blame for having been ill at an inappropriate time that was challenging not only for her but for those charged with her care. While Helen went on to say that she does in fact have a wide circle of close friends, the fundamental problem of trust seems central to her life and also apparently linked to life stage in that she feels she could not have expected friends at the age of 17 to have stood by her. They moved on and she felt 'different', separated from her peer group by cancer at a crucial point in her life trajectory. However, Ashley felt that intervention could break the cycle and help survivors move on:

People will hang onto their disease in a way that can be very unhealthy to them. And the way to deal with that is ... to look the monster in the face, and understand it, and move on and live a life free of the condition, as much as they possibly can ... But that very often needs intervention. It needs positive intervention. A third party can be very useful, somebody who's not caught up in the whole process. Somebody at the end of a helpline for example who can take a completely fresh perspective, and give an input that is new and different, and designed to break a cycle of behaviour.

(Ashley: 37 yrs after diagnosis with CTCL)

However, Maz was clearly accessing psychological support that did not appear to have been entirely successful for him:

I got really bad depression problem and that's why I have to take the pills, for depression. And I'm going to see after every 2 months ... you know a psychologist ... at the hospital. Going there and just to talk to him and whatever he ... say 'you do this and you do that', that's what I'm trying to do you see. That's the only way I know that I need to get help with this life, but I can't do that really well. Sometimes [I'm] fed up, sometimes I can't control my angerness and it's true ... That's why I try to hurt myself ... I don't want to do that but I can't control my feelings you see, because [I'm] fed up.

(Maz: 4 yrs after diagnosis with Ewing's sarcoma)

We have already seen in Chapter 3 that Majad had a profound fear of recurrence and this manifested itself in what seems to be an emotional fragility that comes through in the following quote:

I don't ... well if like recently I've been getting pains in my stomach, in my chest and in my back ... only one thing in my head is I think it's going to come back, I think it's going to back. Because when I were going through it ... when I were going through the pain before I got diagnosed, the pain was in my stomach, in my back for a good 6 months. Before I got diagnosed it was 6 months and after. And [both] my legs, they went numb on me. So that's when they found out I got stomach cancer. And before that you know, for 6 months/7 months I was just on tablets and you know what not and everything. But that's what made me go you know, a bit loopy in the head, because like for 7 months I was on drugs you know, which weren't helping. And for 7 months I was going through that pain which nobody can go through, I swear it. You know like I've been through it, and I know I've been through it. And I know what the pain was to me, because it was in me you know. And it was really terrible you know, because I couldn't sleep, I couldn't walk, I couldn't eat, I couldn't do anything.

(Majad: 7 yrs after his original diagnosis with testicular cancer)

Majad left the interview after about half an hour to move his car, he said that his wife, Rizwana, knew everything about him and would continue talking to me. Once he had left the room she said the following:

Once he's in that state of mind thinking oh God I've got the pains, he won't eat, he doesn't sleep, he doesn't even want to talk, he doesn't socialise, he doesn't do anything. He just wants to be on his own. And I mean like because he smokes as well you see, so he'll be like smoking every 5 minutes. If he's in a good day he won't even ... you hardly, hardly see him having a cigarette ... he won't let go of it [smoking] ... he's tried so many times to give up, and he just won't stop. He won't stop. But like he was saying, like what his life was before he had the cancer, he was a totally different person ... he was just so different. Sometimes I look at him now and I think I'd rather him than this one. He was just so different ... not always ... you know paranoid thinking this and that.

(Rizwana: Majad's wife)

Rizwana also told me that Majad had become so depressed he went to his GP for help, and she offered him anti-depressants, but Rizwana was against him accepting the prescription as she feared he would then become dependent on them. It seems as though Rizwana attributes all Majad's emotional problems to the cancer and the effect of this apparent change in personality appears to have had a negative impact on their relationship. In contrast, Jamie acknowledges that although the cancer was not the only reason for his depression it played a big part in it:

There's sort of like a lot of other things that have built up to it over the years. I think the cancer was sort of like the breaking point. It just ... there's so many things went bad and then that happened. And I don't know, it just ... everything just got on top of me. At the moment it's just getting over this depression thing.

(Jamie: 2 yrs after diagnosis with testicular cancer)

It seems difficult for Jamie to separate the causes of his depression, but the cancer diagnosis appears to have contributed significantly. While Rowena had not experienced depression as a result of her (two) cancers, her illnesses had caused her to become intolerant of the trivial illness of others:

I don't suffer fools gladly anymore ... obviously everybody gets ill from time to time, but I always try and say well you're not ill really. You've just got a cold. You've just got this ... I've gone through something really bad ... But I don't suffer fools gladly now when they say that they're ill. Whether it's close family, or whether it's people at work, I'm very hard on people.

(Rowena: 12 yrs after first diagnosis with Hodgkin's lymphoma)

The term 'suffer fools gladly' was also used by Mary who seems to have adopted a very similar outlook to Rowena:

I can be very demanding. I'm very demanding of myself, and I'm quite demanding of other people. That's not altogether a bad thing, but it can

be a bit much I think. And I don't suffer fools very gladly. I can be pretty
short tempered.

(Mary: 24 yrs after diagnosis with Hodgkin's lymphoma)

Trevor had experienced relatively few negative consequences after his illness;
he appeared to view his cancer with equanimity and was measured in his
responses, so in some ways I was surprised that towards the end of the interview he said the following:

The only ... negative memory, was kind of walking into the hospital, and
the smell of hospitals just in general would bring on an almost physical
sickness – you know purely mentally stimulated, of the hospital and association and everything else. But you know that used to be kind of horrible ... I had treatment every time I went in there, so I went in with a
handkerchief soaked in aftershave or something to disguise the smell ...
Even if we went to see people in hospital, when I wasn't going in for treatment or a check-up, it was almost the same thing. Just the smell of hospitals brought back a lot of, probably fairly ... fairly horrible memories.

(Trevor: 24 yrs after diagnosis with Hodgkin's lymphoma)

While Trevor indicated that this phenomenon had been reduced after about
5 or 6 years, the strength of his response to smell clearly denotes a lasting
emotional connection to a traumatic period in his life. It also adds weight to
the accounts in the last chapter about the emotional impact of attending
follow-up clinics.

Risk taking

As we saw in the first chapter, Cox *et al.* (2005) suggest that survivors of
cancer frequently practice high-risk behaviours. Adolescence and young
adulthood is a time when risk-taking behaviour manifests under ordinary
circumstances as part of the separation from dependence on parents and
the quest for autonomy and individuality (Grinyer 2002a, 2007). Combining
the two effects of adolescent risk-taking and post-cancer survivorship risk-
taking, raises the question of whether it is more likely that survivors of
adolescent cancer will take risks. There is some evidence from the participants that this might be the case. However, the way in which this is played out
may be unexpected and differ according to personality traits and context. On
the one hand the experience of cancer can lead the young person to be fearful
of taking risks. We have already seen at the start of this chapter that Julie
defines herself as extremely cautious, on the other hand given that the worst
has happened and the young person has survived, a cavalier attitude might
prevail.

Greg's account of his approach to life after cancer illustrates the way in
which 'throwing caution to the wind' can result:

I was always quite heavily risk friendly. I mean at school we were always in trouble and held the record for the most lines done ... that's the years before I was ever ill ... so I was always that sort of person. I think if anything it's only encouraged that side to go further. Arguably there's some sort of, a slight immortality complex can develop I think ... it's impacted on the way that you would approach certain things. You might have approached certain things with a little bit more restraint or, or fear or, or respect if it wasn't for the fact that you have this sort of feeling that it doesn't matter. You know ... everything will be fine. You know you'll be okay.

But I guess so much happened, so, so many sort of terrible bits of news and then, and then all these big things, through absolutely no cause of your own ... and I've never really thought about this before ... but subconsciously you can only think well, you know I'm always going to be okay. It doesn't really matter, there's no clear reason why. So something was cured and it came back, and it was cured and it came back, and, and then it was cured and why do all these things, every time anything seems to happen I always seem to be able to get up and walk away still ... You wouldn't think oh yes ... I can do anything, I'll be fine. But there's certainly an element of that I think. Particularly I think when you're coming out of it aged sort of 16, 17 where I think boys of that age are prone to those sort of thoughts anyway aren't they? I had a bit of a descent for about 8 years in terms of what I did, drinking, smoking, drug taking etcetera, that sort of thing.

(Greg: 19 yrs after diagnosis with osteosarcoma)

Interestingly, Greg attributes his risk-taking behaviour to an apparently residual feeling of invincibility; after all he survived not just one relapse but several, as he was diagnosed with lung secondaries from his osteosarcoma on more than one occasion. Nevertheless, we cannot ignore his admission of a previous tendency to take risks from an early age. Perhaps what is more surprising is that after having had sections of lung removed on several occasions during his illness when secondaries were diagnosed, he now smokes:

Smoking is one that I've always looked at differently to everything else. It is the one that I've always felt I shouldn't do. Whereas I'm never really concerned about [anything] else that I've done. But that doesn't mean I'll ever stop doing it, just that I'll be okay ... you know I tried, I've been giving up for the last 5 years now because my daughter's 5 ... and I've successfully given up during the day, it's just if I drink or anything like that though. And that's the instant that it, that it sort of kicks in, the desire to have one. I remember when I first started smoking I thought to myself well I mean everyone else might get addicted but I won't do ... but it's the approach that I take to most things where you sort of take all facts and then remove them to the side and just have your own opinion based on what you want to do on that day. And it's an easy decision to, to make.

(Greg: 19 yrs after diagnosis with osteosarcoma)

Of course we cannot remove the element of addiction to nicotine from Greg's decision to smoke, as clearly at some level he has accepted that it would be better to stop, though it seems that this would be primarily for his daughter's well-being rather than his own. Smoking was raised by both Jamie and Jack as an issue, with Jamie cutting right down and Jack relating the story of a friend who has gone 'too far' by adopting a 'what the hell' attitude:

Smoking-wise … it makes me think well that could have been the reason why I got it in the first place. So it's made me cut down on smoking a lot … the amount that I smoke I might as well quit, because I'll sort of like go 3, 4 weeks without smoking and then I'll smoke for about 2 or 3 days, and then go another 2, 3 weeks without smoking. So it's … I suppose yes, it has made me take care of myself. But I think to myself well if you don't then there's a bigger chance that it's going to come back so … I'm not really a drinker, it's just smoking that it's really made me cut down on really.

(Jamie: 2 yrs after diagnosis with testicular cancer)

I'd say I'm definitely more likely to take a risk. But I have a friend of mine who went through a similar treatment … he went too far with it. He kind of just thought well if this is going to happen to me then I might as well smoke 40 cigarettes a day, and he's an alcoholic, and just went off the scales. So it kind of … and I'm sure some people can go either way really. Some people can lock themselves inside, and some people can throw caution to the wind.

(Jack: 9 yrs after diagnosis with Hodgkin's lymphoma)

The legacy of the illness for Dan has been to raise his awareness of health-related lifestyle and healthy choices perhaps unusual in this age group:

I'm much more aware of diet and lifestyle. And I don't think … I suppose that might sound a bit silly but I drink quite a lot of green tea and that sort of thing, you know anti-oxidants. And I do things that generally wouldn't put my health at risk. You know I have loads of really early nights, and I've made lifestyle changes I suppose … it's not really in response to a bad lifestyle before but it's just more that I'm more aware now … I never, ever drink to excess or anything like that. And you know I think it very possibly has made me a bit safe if you like.

(Dan: 5 yrs after diagnosis with testicular cancer)

In contrast Huxley relates his craving for risk to the adrenaline release he believes to have been associated with his chemotherapy:

I never, never liked huge adrenaline releases. I was never a person to get on a motorbike and ride fast or go white-water rafting or ... I loved sport [but] there was a control involved – it was a field and a ball and the rules are pretty simple and if you're good at it you can stick to it. I love swimming because it's up and down a pool. They were the things that I liked ... but a lot of the chemicals that they put through your system when you're having chemotherapy, give you massive adrenaline releases. Just through the sort of like the chemical changes that they put into your body. So ever since then it changed the way ... I actually looked upon experiences. And there was something that I was craving as such. And fairground rides, jumping out of planes, you know bungee jumping whatever – if someone were to offer it to me I'd say 'definitely'. So do you know I've done all the mad fairground rides, and if someone says, 'Oh come and do this' I'll say 'Yes, definitely and let's have a go.' So that's just because all of that natural adrenaline release is a really, really comforting feeling. Do you know what I mean, whether it's you're that scared for a minute, feeling normal is great – I don't know. And that was ... definitely brought on with the cancer experience I would have said, yes ... it made me a lot more adventurous as a person. And yes we've had some really, really great times in the last sort of 17 years, 18 years of my life, so yes it's been good.

(Huxley: 18 yrs after diagnosis with ALL)

However, even if Huxley had come to need the adrenaline rush of risk-taking activities, his attitude to foods had become much more cautious. As he said 'I was the mixed grill king, I'd eat anything you put in front of me ... it didn't bother me.' Yet as a result of his illness his diet had changed for the better as he said: 'Massively, massively, yes, and all my family.'

Later in this chapter we look at the way in which philosophy and approach to life has been shaped by the cancer experience, but pre-empt it here with this comment from Vicky:

I guess it's made me take more risks. Want to do more things, see more things ... if there's any opportunity of doing something I'll do it. You know if there's any ... if someone says ... a group of my female friends for example 'shall we go to Barcelona?', you know I won't even think twice about it, I'll just do it ... probably because I just think that after everything I went through I'm extremely lucky to be here. But you know the fertility aside, and I just want to live every moment I guess.

(Vicky: 5 yrs after diagnosis with ovarian cancer)

Seizing the moment seemed to have been the motivation for some of Paul's risk-taking behaviour:

Maybe not so much now, but definitely there was a peak of sort of like yes, more risk-taking. More risk ... you know because one, you know they might … they … you know may … the next I go see them they may say well you must come back in another 3 months. I'd also prepared myself for the fact that this could go on and on. And then to be liked ripped back … for a while I was thinking I could get pulled back in at any point so yes the risk-taking definitely I think. I did stupid things that I would never have … well I say stupid things but … I got sort of like a bit of a reputation of like you know … I can remember once, this is just a stupid one. We were going into town, sort of from where we lived, like a group of lads. And there wasn't enough room, we we're going to have to get a taxi, but I mean we were all students, we couldn't really afford it. And then there was room in the boot … and everyone [was] like, 'Oh Paul will go in the boot like.' Oh I've never done that before, you know what I'm off in the boot, you know rattling along and just for the sort of … just sort of experience. Not that it's particularly dangerous, but you know I got sort of a reputation of if there's something different Paul will try it.

> (Paul: 9 yrs after diagnosis with testicular cancer)

Julie identified herself as a cautious person yet she acknowledges that when first diagnosed with Hodgkin's lymphoma she felt the need to take chances in a way that was uncharacteristic for her:

Well definitely when I did have that first diagnosis, it does make you realise how precious life is. And that I wanted to go and experience a whole load of things I hadn't experienced before. So I sort of had made a list, and did all sorts of maniac things. I don't know, not that maniac, just sort of things I hadn't done before, I don't know … being more risky. I don't know just stupid things like I went white-water rafting. And I mean some people do those sorts of things all the time, but for me that's unusual. And, I don't know, went out in somebody's speedboat. And, oh I don't know, loads of different things … it wasn't that I saw it as a challenge, I saw it as an opportunity I think. As to just, you know, do things I hadn't done before, and just value things more.

> (Julie:15 yrs after first diagnosis with Hodgkin's lymphoma)

Julie also told me that just before her mastectomy for a later breast cancer she wanted to do a 'Thelma and Louise' that is to 'flash' her breasts – while she still had the opportunity. She managed this on a canal barge and seemed gratified that she had summoned the courage taken the risk. Both Andrea and Lesley adopted a selective approach to risk-taking:

[I'm a] risk taker, maybe in some terms but not in others. I mean I'm not one to sort of maybe take risks with money or that sort of thing you know. But yes, I tend to think that maybe one day I'll do a parachute jump and that sort of thing. Whether I ever will or not you know, I do have these little you know. That sort of thing as far as risk-taking, I do think I would be more inclined ... I think it's ... I think it's a thing I have of having an experience. I don't want to miss out on that experience in life.

(Andrea: 21 yrs after diagnosis with acute myeloid leukaemia)

I don't know whether I take more or less risks, because I know some people, like friends, will talk to me and think I do take risks in that I've changed my job quite a few times, we've moved house ... we moved house about 6 times in 12 years I think at one stage. And I do go for things. But I think I feel that that would have been me anyway. And then in some ways I think myself that I don't take as many risks in.

(Lesley: 18 yrs after diagnosis with Hodgkin's lymphoma)

Elaine B had been a professional skater who, it could be argued, had taken physical risks in her professional life, yet she had adopted a much more cautious approach to her skating in what appears to be a very pragmatic and practical assessment of the risks to her now more fragile bones, but she also speaks of having more fear in her:

If anything I would say slightly less risks ... with skating now, I won't try and do things that I used to be able to do, because of falling. My bones are weaker. [A result of the illness] yes, osteoporosis ... they were weak bones ... I don't think I'd risk falling over ... I think I've got more fear in me now ... I wouldn't try things like bungee jumping, or something that could damage your health.

(Elaine B: 15 yrs after diagnosis with Hodgkin's lymphoma)

Marc is the only participant to have drawn a distinction between risk and challenge, and for him the challenges have become a lifestyle choice:

I'm not sure that I should call it risk, but I think I'm certainly more challenge orientated. So I think there's a slight difference there. I don't want to do something where I'm likely to kill myself; that to me is risk. Where a challenge is something different, where I'll put obstacles in front of myself that are going to be difficult to achieve, I'm not going to kill myself doing it but ... so I've become a challenge junkie, but I wouldn't say I was a risk junkie.

(Marc: 21 yrs after diagnosis with osteosarcoma)

Philosophy of life

The experience of life-threatening illness has long-lasting and far-reaching effects on the life of the survivor long after the illness is over and can shape attitudes towards how a life 'should' be lived. Discussing illness narratives, Frank argues that these expressions of the experience 'claim that the illness has helped the author to discover the point of his or her own life' (2002: 169).

Zebrack and Chesler make a similar comment that the necessity of facing up to a life-threatening illness can inspire people to live in a different way and 'can provide clarification about what and who is truly important to them' (in Langeveld and Arbuckle 2008: 149). Seizing the moment and experiencing all life has to offer underlie some of the accounts of risk-or challenge-taking provided earlier. Does this mean that a fundamental change to survivors' philosophy of life has taken place? Some of the following accounts suggest that this is indeed the case.

Louise commented on her changed attitude to life beginning with some examples of risk-taking:

> I've jumped out of a plane in Australia; I've climbed Sydney Harbour Bridge ... I've been on lots of holidays, had a baby, got engaged. I've got a good job ... I guess life's too short. The thing is for me that I was a survivor and right from the beginning ... I mean I had the lump growing out my back. And then after the first dose of chemo my lump started to go down. So I reacted really, really quickly ... but at the same time when I went through my second part of my chemo after my operation, my aunt got ill with secondary breast cancer ... as I was getting better she was getting worse. And she had all the side effects that ... and all the horrible things that come with secondary breast cancer. And so I saw the worst side of what cancer can do, like for her. So it's just made me think right, life's too short.
> (Louise: 8 yrs after diagnosis with Ewing's sarcoma)

For Louise her approach to life seems to have been shaped not only by her own cancer experience but also by the contrasting outcome of her aunt's cancer, thus throwing into relief her good fortune at being a survivor. In the following quotation, Kirsty actually says that it has changed her philosophy:

> When I first got diagnosed I thought to myself oh you know, well maybe this was ... like you know maybe this was my fate, and all of this. But then I thought you know, I think things like oh you know people believe in karma, and fate, and all of this. And I just thought well actually I like really don't believe in that anymore, because you know if karma's true and things like that then you know what have I done ... so bad ... I think it's definitely something that's played in the back of my head that perhaps you know it's something that I wasn't ... you know I wasn't supposed to fulfil my whole life. So now I definitely think well I shall. And I'll have a good time doing it, and enjoy it while it lasts kind of thing ... I just think well you know, live each day as it comes kind of thing. Whereas before I was constantly planning you know. I decided I had my life plan – I was going to university, and then I was off to get a job. And you know, and then I just thought well whatever comes my way now, it comes my way. And you know I do a lot more things that perhaps I wouldn't have done before, and try and experience things like that. Because I suppose an

element of me probably is quite sort of you know, aware of the fact that my cancer could come back. And you know I don't want to regret anything. So I think definitely it has changed my philosophy on sort of my life now going forward.

(Kirsty: 5 yrs after diagnosis with Hodgkin's lymphoma)

In a very similar vein Katie says:

It's made me sort of appreciate things a lot more ... I always used to worry a little bit about dying early. You know dying young, or my husband dying young. I think it's made me more aware that that can happen. Because I think you're just going to assume oh that sort of thing you read about it but it happens to other people, it doesn't happen to me. And I think very early on in my adult life I was reminded that actually that could happen to me. And I think that's always going to be with me, the knowledge that you can't just assume that I'm going to live to 80 or whatever.

(Katie: 13 yrs after diagnosis with ovarian cancer)

While Katie has a strong sense that 'anything could happen' and that it is not only people you read about who experience tragedy, she nevertheless seems to have an enhanced appreciation of life that is no longer taken for granted. The essence of this approach to life is captured in the following extract from Kelly's account:

I wouldn't take it back for a million pounds. I really wouldn't because ... I feel like I've been given a very privileged opportunity to really be able to value the people around me, and what I have ... it doesn't mean that you don't take things for granted and I quite often get cross with myself because I'll sort of take something for granted and then really wish I hadn't. But I think it gives you that ability to just stop and really appreciate what you've got ... it doesn't change who you are, but it changes how you go about doing things I think, and the thought processes you go through, and how much more deeply you think about things.

(Kelly: 7 yrs after diagnosis with non-Hodgkin's lymphoma)

The fact that nothing can be taken for granted permeated many of the accounts and on the whole rather than leading to feelings of vulnerability resulted in a determination to 'seize the moment', not to be distracted by the trivial, and an intolerance for the unsatisfactory. Although I am not claiming generalisability, I have grouped together a number of quotations that, while varying in detail, all carry some version of this approach to life. I have taken the unusual step of presenting the data *en bloc* in this way as I believe that collectively the similarity has great power. Much of this volume focuses on pain, distress and difficulty, but the message evident from the series of extracts that follow is a very positive one that I believe gains power from the strong resemblance of responses:

My husband's got quite a stressful job. But from my perspective, I don't need that anymore ... I just think you've only got one chance in life. I know I nearly lost it at quite a young age. And I just want to chill really, enjoy the children that I never thought I'd have. I try and live my life just very simply really.

(Lisa: 9 yrs after diagnosis with non-Hodgkin's lymphoma)

In my career I pursue my goals much more ... I'm more interested in succeeding in a relatively short period of time ... and something that I found ... having been ill is that I was more relaxed about trivial things in life, and yet more determined to make the most of life ... when you have a potentially life-threatening illness I think it really focuses the mind. And certainly for me part of that was to sort of make sure that I didn't lose any time if you like.

(Dan: 5 yrs after diagnosis with testicular cancer)

Every now and again you take a stock of what's important to you and what you do with yourself and you know, in times of great joy or pressure you look at yourself in a different way. But you're obviously moulded by your experiences and that's a massive experience to face, at the time was ... sort of could have been death do you know what I mean? So I spent 5 or 6 years just really enjoying the fact that I was alive, do you know what I mean? And yes it's moulded everything that's happened to me since ... I take things as they come. I don't try and plan too far ahead, because you don't know where the future's going to take you ... that's one of the morals that I've lived on ... the fragility of life is brought upon you ... I'm not going to let something stress me out but not do anything about it. It's made me very proactive I think ... The experience has enhanced me as a person I suppose because I've not cheated death as such. I don't look at it as like 'I'm special'. I just look at it as though I'm fortunate and therefore enjoy it while you've got it do you know what I mean? ... You know you cherish your time, so yes it's quite a positive experience really for me.

(Huxley: 18 yrs after diagnosis with ALL)

I think it's changed my perspective on life. I realise that you've got to do things you know, there and then you know rather than wait or 'I'll do it when I've got time' you know. I think now if I decide I want to do something I just go and do it, rather than you know waiting about it.

(Ben: 4 yrs after diagnosis with testicular cancer)

I am aware of how I don't want to waste any time ... and so I have to feel like I'm doing something, and that I'm enjoying sort of things of everyday ... if ever the situation where you're like oh this is a real drag or whatever and you think oh well why am I doing this because you know ... I've thought now that I want to enjoy everyday and I want to feel like everyday is you know, making a difference to me, and hopefully to somebody else … Also you know the sense that anything can happen you know, happen … like you could get run over by a bus, you know but … I really believe it, do you know what I mean?

(Paul: 9 yrs after diagnosis with testicular cancer)

I sort of go through phases of feeling like right what am I doing with my life you know, am I making the most use of it. And he [partner] sort of has to put up with those. And what big things shall we go and do to sort of make sure that, you know I'm sort of fulfilling all that I should do … feeling like well you know, if it all came back again, if I was ill again, then obviously I've sort of wasted this time by not making the most of it.

(Elaine: 5 yrs after diagnosis with Hodgkin's lymphoma)

I always say that yes it has changed my outlook on life. But just to pinpoint exactly why, it's a bit difficult. I think, because being at that age when I was ill, just turning 18, I was very young. And it did make me grow up quite quickly. And I think yes, as far as trying … making the best of everything.

(Andrea: 21 yrs after diagnosis with ALL)

When you come out of that you kind of … you have this … not urgency, but you just have this real different outlook on life to how precious it is, and how everyday's worth so much more than you ever imagined it could be. It's kind of like how fragile life is, and how you need to just grasp every opportunity that comes your way … I don't seem to worry about the little things anymore. I try … well I mean day to day life you still get caught up in everything, but I try and put things in perspective a lot more.

(Phoebe: 2 yrs after diagnosis with acinic cell carcinoma)

I used to worry about absolutely everything when I was younger … but now … the job I've got is a high-pressure job. But everyone always says well you're so chilled … Because I think it's give me that sort of perspective that a lot worse can happen than losing your job. And it doesn't seem to bother me that much, which I don't know if it's a good thing or not … I mean dying is the worst thing that can happen so losing your job's not going to affect that much. So yes, not a lot really affects me that much anymore.

(Paul B: 11 yrs after diagnosis with non-Hodgkin's lymphoma)

It's sort of like I've been given a second chance really and truthfully. So it has made me think that there's a reason for me actually being here before so … because before the operation I thought to myself well I don't know, life's pointless. But when you come through something like that it just ... it makes you look at life in a totally different way so ... I don't know, you have to be scared into things really and truthfully, until you stop taking things for granted.

(Jamie: 2 yrs after diagnosis with testicular cancer)

I vowed then I'd never, ever stay working somewhere where I wasn't happy ... I'm very relaxed, I'm very laid back, I don't get upset about little things, because you know in the grand scheme of things it really isn't important. I feel terribly, terribly grateful to be here, really thankful for my children – really, really thankful for the opportunities that I've got ... I'm not a religious person, and I didn't you know, turn to God or anything like that. But something about me definitely changed with the illness. Again I think that maybe having been a) so frightened, and b) so vulnerable, and then as the treatment progressed, so really poorly by the end of it, I think you've only got to think back on those days and realise that actually you know, things today really aren't bad at all ... There's something very cathartic about the whole thing, definitely.

(Debbie: 22 yrs after diagnosis with Hodgkin's lymphoma)

It's certainly changed my outlook. I don't tend to sort of get hung up on the small unimportant things I think anymore ... You know I used to sort of really preoccupy myself with small details and sort of have sleepless nights, and you know things like that. You know completely unimportant things. But now, you know it just sort of washes straight over my head and you know I pick up on the important things ... now I'm just easy come, easy go, you know take things with a pinch of salt.

(Michael: 5 yrs after diagnosis with testicular cancer)

I decided that I wanted to try and make the most of whatever time I did have left. So I didn't know what this diagnosis meant, and what my prognosis really was going to be. I didn't know how long I was going to survive, but I wanted to make sure that if I was going to do something in the time that I had left, I was going to do it to the best of my ability. And even though it's a long time ago since I had all my cancer, I still keep that in my mind that if I'm going to do something I want to do it to the best of my ability ... it did make me really focus on how I wanted to live my life, and at a kind of critical time when you do make decisions about how you want to be.

(Marc: 21 yrs after diagnosis with osteosarcoma)

For me as an individual I think it certainly – as again many cancer survivors say – it certainly gave me a new perspective on life. You know you do tend to appreciate life that little bit more. But you know, there is not a day goes by, because I know how fortunate that I am ... my philosophy is live life to the full, enjoy it while you can, because life is not a rehearsal. There is no second chance to enjoy it.

(John: 33 yrs after diagnosis with Hodgkin's lymphoma)

I mean you value milestones in your life. From my point of view I valued my 21st. But more so I valued my 40th, because I felt I've got this far, who'd have thought if they'd have seen me in Christies in 1981, that I would be here celebrating my 40th birthday with my two girls who they thought I wouldn't have. And this year I'm celebrating my silver wedding with my husband who was my boyfriend/fiancé at the time. But it makes you appreciate that you've got to those milestones really.

(Janet: 27 yrs after diagnosis with Hodgkin's lymphoma)

Summary

Once again readers may ask what life stage has to do with this chapter? Does surviving adolescent and young adult cancer really carry with it a different quality of emotional impact than survival from cancer at other life stages? I suspect that this chapter is the one with least explicit evidence of life stage as a defining factor. Nevertheless, the aim of the research was to understand the long-term impact and examine what survivorship means. Even if the accounts presented here may not be distinctive in age-related terms, what they demonstrate is that however long it has been since the cancer diagnosis and treatment, the emotional impact – for good and ill – is lasting. It can shape life, attitudes and choices.

Soliman and Agresta argue that the effects of cancer for this age group can vary from life-affirming experiences to tribulations that cause hopelessness and despair (2008: 59). This is borne out by the contradictions evident in this chapter – from the contrast between the emotional legacy resulting in feelings of vulnerability and symptoms akin to PTS, through to the quotes provided all of which indicate a reordering of priorities and a change in perspective that suggest that life is viewed as a gift not to be taken for granted, not to be wasted, to be appreciated and lived fully at all times.

The approach to risk-taking again shows some contradiction, there are clearly those who take greater risks, in part to maximise experience and in part as an act of defiance. However there are also those who have become cautious or even manifest a combination of risk aversion and risk-taking. It is impossible to say with certainty that these differential approaches to risk-taking are a heightened form of previous character traits but the implication is – according to participants like Greg – that this is the case and that rather than changing a person's character, pre-existing tendencies are accentuated. It is not within the remit of this research to offer a psychological analysis or explanation; nevertheless, it seems clear that whatever the emotional impact it has a lasting effect, though this may change in nature over a period of time and be triggered by other life events.

The risks addressed in the interviews were confined largely to the socially acceptable and legal; but as Levitt and Eshelman say data regarding for example, illicit drug use, are scarce in the survivor population as they are confounded by self-report bias (2008: 181). Even the degree of trust and rapport I was able to establish with participants was unlikely to result in confessions of illegal activity and in fact only one young man admitted to such risk-taking.

So what effect does the life stage during the illness have on the long-term emotional impact? There are few explicit comments on the effect of age at diagnosis; nevertheless there are some embedded indications that it was significant. For example, problems with trust that manifested after friends failed to sustain support were reported by Helen, and this does seem to be a function of age and life stage during the illness. The effect of a life being interrupted at a pivotal stage may account for the tendency to 'seize the moment', and not letting any more time or opportunities pass by. But on the negative side, the shock of a cancer diagnosis at a time in life when it is so unexpected can leave lasting feelings of vulnerability that permeate relationships, shape attitudes and result in concerns and fears, for example for the health and well-being of future generations.

It is arguable that cancer diagnosed earlier in childhood may be left behind to a greater extent and cancer diagnosed in later life is neither so unusual nor does it occur at such a formative and unexpected moment. It is also apparent that the range of time since diagnosis in no sense seems to have mitigated the quality of the responses. The power of the recollection and emotions appears undiluted even after many years have elapsed. This observation comes not only from the words uttered by the participants but from my engagement with them, the way in which they recollected the experience and the emotions apparent during the interviews.

Soliman and Agresta (2008) suggest that susceptibility to major psychiatric illness in survivors is not solely related to their cancer history and it seems from the testimonies provided that this is indeed the case. However, Soliman and Agresta do claim that regular assessment and appropriate treatment is needed by this age group who may experience chronic medical issues or difficulty in attaining their life goals.

Key points

Emotional impact

* Feelings of vulnerability
* Fearing the worst
* Post Traumatic Stress (PTS)
* Lack of trust in others and the future

Risk taking

* Risks taken in order to relish experience and celebrate life
* Risks taken out of a sense of immortality
* Risks avoided to protect fragile health
* Risks avoided to limit further stress

Philosophy of life

* Nothing taken for granted
* Trivial concerns were dismissed
* Opportunities welcomed and grasped
* Unwillingness to tolerate unsatisfactory situations
* Awareness of mortality heighted appreciation of life

6 Survivorship identity, the resistance to victimhood and the positive outcomes

McKenzie and Crouch utilise Giddens' concept of identity as a starting point for their discussion of survivorship. They argue that the customary conventions of human discourse are vulnerable to being undermined by an event such as cancer and that the resulting mantle of uncertainty and risk can appear as 'unwelcome omens of hazard' (2004: 142); voicing fears may be discouraged and cancer survivorship identity may need to be subsumed to resume 'normal' relationships. They claim that 'Not only do cancer survivors feel isolated in their pain, but their very identities – indelibly inscribed by the cancer experience – are pushed to the margins of the social fabric in which selfhood is embedded' (McKenzie and Crouch 2004: 143).

However, in contrast to an assumed need to subsume the survivorship identity, Lance Armstrong, a survivor of testicular cancer, not only survived to win the Tour de France, but also to write his autobiography focusing on his illness and recovery, and interpreted his cancer as something he had been given 'for the good of others'. As a result he founded a Charitable Foundation and is quoted as saying: 'Maybe my role was to be a cancer survivor' (2000: 155–156). Frank (2002) commenting on Armstrong's construction of his identity as a survivor argues that here 'survivor' means much more than simply having remained alive, it means that he has a mission (2002: 169).

Frank cites Armstrong's oncologist as describing him as having 'the obligation of the cured' (2002: 170). This suggests that those who survive an illness, in this case cancer, survive with some degree of responsibility to aid others who experience it. There is also an implication that an element of gratitude should be felt for the survival and that there is a concomitant 'duty' to repay the 'debt'. However, to do so requires the survivor to take on the identity of 'cancer survivor'. Mathieson and Stam (1995) suggest that living with cancer is identity-altering. It situates the individual within the context of organised social relationships and inscribes the disease into their biography; this is made clear in Elizabeth Bryan's account of her cancer:

> Meanwhile I am struggling to re-establish my identity and role. Who am I now? For more than 30 years I was a paediatrician and specialist in

twins and triplets. Last year I was a cancer sufferer and invalid. Now I am no longer an invalid nor am I an interesting case at the hospital.

(Bryan 2008: 5)

If Bryan's well-established identity in her professional role can be so undermined by her illness, identity crisis may be even more acute for those whose illness was diagnosed and treated at an age and life stage when other identities are fragile (Grinyer 2002a). Langeveld and Arbuckle say that in the transition from patient to survivor, young people must establish a new identity that incorporates their cancer but does not define them (2008: 150).

This volume looks at survivorship in the longer-term, thus it may be that the willingness or otherwise to take on the mantle of 'survivor' and accept this as part of one's identity changes as time progresses. We saw in Chapter 4, that while not feeling the need for a support group themselves, some participants indicated that they would find it gratifying to help others – thus in Frank's (2002) terms taking up the 'obligation of the cured' and implicitly accepting 'survivorship identity'.

However, Jacobs (1985) argues that the identity achieved during adolescence and young adulthood is not necessarily life-long and that further adult development refines identity. Yet Jacobs also suggests that if young people are 'labelled' they can react badly and may well carry that label with them through life in a way that shapes future interactions. If the perception of adolescents and young adults with cancer is that, at a crucial moment in the identity formation period, they have been labelled 'patient' or 'cancer sufferer' then there is a risk that this will impede further development and the emergence of other more positive identities.

Survivorship identity

Dan, who by the time of my interview with him had made a successful career as an artist, had considerable ambivalence about his survivorship identity. Much of his early artwork had represented his cancer experience. The artwork he presented for his degree, charted his cancer journey through powerful depictions of the stages through which he had been:

> I've completed that body of work ... once I'd done those paintings I felt that I had completed it and I was ready to move on ... I had to present it for university and so that finished the chapter in a way ... I certainly would never revisit my work on my cancer experience. I wouldn't want to; I would have no interest in doing so at all ... I was very much defined as ... the 'cancer victim' or 'survivor' who did art on it and then in art circles I was the artist who'd had cancer. To some extent that will go on. But actually to be honest I'd much prefer to be known as an artist ... not long after my treatment finished if I ever met anyone new I would introduce myself and would have this real urge to tell them that I'd been ill and that

I'd had cancer. And I'd just somehow manage to slip it into conversation you know. I'd just manage to turn the conversation round to say, 'Oh yes I've ...' you know 'I've had testicular cancer.' And then I started to recognise that actually that wasn't very healthy. And so actually I almost made myself not do that you know. And putting that behind me has almost enabled me to go on as myself rather than as defined by my illness. Because my illness really was only 6 months out of my life ... well a bit longer. But you know it wasn't such a long time, although it was quite an intense period ... [There was an] article on me on the cancer artwork soon after I did it ... it was about me being ill and doing the artwork and so on. And now [there] is a follow-up article but about my current business. And I haven't seen the copy yet, but it will mention my illness, because in that instance it has to in order to get the story out. So part of me does think, 'yes I do want to be known as an artist yes' and I am still happy to talk about my experience for the benefit of others, but I don't want to come across as vulnerable really anymore ... you don't want people to think that you're just making it because you were ill and you've got the sympathy vote. You know I want to make it, and, 'Oh by the way I also had cancer.' I want to be more like Lance Armstrong in that respect ... I don't mind people knowing at all. But I want to be known for my skills and talent more than for overcoming adversity.

(Dan: 5 yrs after diagnosis with testicular cancer)

Dan raises many issues in this quotation – it seems significant that he actively wishes to move away from a position in which he is defined by his illness history, yet he acknowledges that to some extent this was an identity he embraced in the early stages. The comment Dan makes about Lance Armstrong is particularly interesting as Armstrong (2000) states that his role as a cancer survivor is in fact integral to his identity and he alludes to the belief that this is what the experience of having had cancer was 'for'. Yet Dan clearly interprets Armstrong's post-cancer activities predominantly as a sportsman not as a survivor, and having made clear his own resistance to being labelled a 'survivor' actually cites Armstrong as a 'role model' for his own professional versus survivorship identity. It is also clear that Dan is resistant to any portrayal that would make him appear 'vulnerable' and this is a theme that we return to later in this chapter.

Thomas identified himself as a survivor but was ambivalent about the extent to which he had adopted this role as part of his identity. He too, like Dan, disliked strongly any resonance of victimhood:

I mean on one level it's [identity] having no hair, and that's now a permanent thing because of the amount of radiotherapy ... I can't actually imagine myself with hair ... and all the weight and the body shape changes and things like that ... I find [it] hard relate to the person in the photograph when I was a kid [as me]. But it's also I think how other people perceive me. I worry that ... people think of me as Tom the guy who had cancer, or survived cancer ... that word 'victim' ... I'm not happy with that word being used ... I was just looking at some stuff and it said 'Tom who's spoken to some other victims', it's not very nice ... I think also there's a little bit of denial on my part of wanting that label of the person who survived cancer, and so I don't want to get too involved with those people [other survivors] I want to have regular friends as well.

(Thomas: 13 yrs after diagnosis with a brain tumour)

It seems from Thomas' reflections that not only does he not wish to be defined by his survivorship; he does not wish to be ghettoised by it. Yet Thomas is someone who has spoken of his experience at conferences and who has acted as an advocate for other young adult patients. Nevertheless, he is a young man who primarily wishes to be regarded as 'normal' and to associate with 'regular' friends.

In contrast, John, much longer after his cancer, identified strongly as a survivor and has written a self-published book about his experience. He also has a website devoted to his cancer experience that aims to 'provide hope and inspiration to anyone affected by a cancer diagnosis' (www.johnwpattison. com) but he emphasised that though his survivorship informed his professional interactions as a nurse with cancer patients, he would not divulge this identity to them:

It is part of my identity without question ... it manifests itself in my daily life purely and simply with my, you know my nursing career, which as I say is of paramount importance to me, because it allows me to give something back, and to you know to help other cancer patients and survivors. But no, I wouldn't go out of my way to tell [patients] deliberately.

(John: 33 yrs after diagnosis with Hodgkin's lymphoma)

So, like Bob, John is putting something back into the system, not because he had a bad experience as a patient, but possibly as a manifestation of the 'duty of the cured'. Louise, had identified herself as a cancer survivor in an article she had written for a national newspaper, similar to Ruth's use of the web-based account of her cancer (Chapter 2), Louise used this article as a device to tell her new boyfriend (who later became her fiancé) about her cancer:

I'd done an article for *The Telegraph* quite a few years ago. And I think it was on like our second or our third date I showed him some of my articles that I'd done ... like 'My Life as Cancer Patient' ... and I just showed him that. And he just went through the article, and it really made like just think oh you know, I'm really glad I've got you sort of thing. It was really nice. And then I was quite paranoid obviously about him seeing my back. But it didn't affect him at all, it really didn't.

(Louise: 8 yrs after diagnosis with Ewing's sarcoma)

It seems that Louise introduced her cancer survivorship identity in stages – firstly the written account and subsequently the manifestation of the physical legacy – again part of her 'identity' but difficult to disclose. Kelly's confidence at social occasions had been affected negatively since her cancer; she found it difficult to walk into a room full of people if there was not a 'real purpose' for her to be there – as if her presence alone were not enough. Some of Kelly's insecurity in her identity came from the fact that because of her illness she had not been able to engage fully in the usual teenage activities and felt that this had set her apart from her peers and that even 7 years later she had not caught up. However, Kelly had become involved in charitable work related to teenage cancer; this had conferred identity and given her a defined role:

> I would find it very difficult to walk into a pub on my own [but] if I'm doing something for the charity and I walk into a charity event I feel fine, because I feel like I'm kind of justified in being there, and I've got a purpose … I feel that I can say anything and nobody can turn round to me and tell me that I'm wrong, because it's my experience … I've been involved in the charity since before I finished my treatment, so they're a group of people who know me. So I'm not just there as a professional survivor, I'm there because I've done my dissertation to do with the charity as well. So … [I] feel like I've got something to say that's worthwhile, and that the people who are there know that it's worthwhile. So it's not just about being a survivor, it's about feeling valued in that setting.
>
> But I find that if friends invite me to go out, you know not so much to the pub but you know out into town or something like that, 9 times out of 10 I'll say yes but I won't go … I think it has got to do with how I perceive myself, and a lack of confidence in sort of where I fit in, and who I'll talk to, and what I'll talk about.
>
> (Kelly: 7 yrs after diagnosis with non-Hodgkin's lymphoma)

It seems that Kelly has adopted a secure identity as a survivor – and an authoritative survivor who has completed academic work for her degree on the topic – yet this confidence has not extended to the wider social environment. However, Kelly's compulsion to tell everyone she met about her cancer has receded over the years:

> When I met people I felt like I had to say, 'Hi, I'm Kelly … I've had cancer.' And that was almost the most important thing about me, so it was something that I felt that I really needed to tell people about myself to almost justify who I was. And I don't feel that anymore.
>
> (Kelly, 7 yrs after diagnosis with non-Hodgkin's lymphoma)

So far all the participants in this chapter had 'gone public' to some extent, and so had Greg, but to friends rather than in print, through charitable involvement or on the Internet. On the subject of taking on the identity of a cancer survivor

Greg concurs with Dan and Kelly that this changes over time, nevertheless while the feeling about identity may change the physical legacy may not:

> I think that changes over time. I think it certainly was to start with ... very much probably was to start with. I mean I can swing my arm round this way because it's not connected properly, and I used to do that all the time. Just go, just for entertainment value and to ... get drinks off people and so on. I think it was probably more part of my identity before university to be honest ... and the older I get the, the less I want to be associated with it altogether. I guess that you'd be quite happily proud of the scars. It's something that's yours to make you different I guess. And it's something that you know you can be proud of, and that you would probably show people perhaps deliberately. But I don't think that lasts for very long.
>
> (Greg: 19 yrs after diagnosis with osteosarcoma)

Greg raises the notion of pride in his survivorship and this relates to Katie's resistance to being identified as a victim; indeed she suggests that the very word 'survivor' can be positive:

> I'm very determined not to be a victim ... one of the funny, quirky things that's come out of it is that ... from when I had the cancer I've hated the words like 'victim', 'brave' you know that you get in the newspapers and things like that. Just because I thought, well I don't see myself as a victim. I'm just a person who happens to be ill ... certainly the word 'victim' is a very disempowering word and I didn't feel like that ... I don't want to be seen like that and it ... still annoys me when you see it in the papers you know this little child, 'oh cancer victim, brave and all this' ... [The term survivor is] fine, because to me that's a fairly neutral word. You know it's something you had and it could have killed you but it didn't. I think survivor's a fairly neutral, sometimes a positive word ... and as I say I don't like 'victim' just because I feel it is quite disempowering, quite a negative sort of word. It makes someone seem weak which I think well I wasn't weak, I just happened to be ill.
>
> (Katie: 13 yrs after diagnosis with ovarian cancer)

I interviewed Kate 31 years after her diagnosis yet it seems that the strength of her feeling about her identity as a survivor and her abhorrence of being seen as a 'sufferer' or 'victim' have not dimmed with the passing years, indeed she still has a strong resistance to the term 'patient':

> It's being cancer-free has made me a survivor, otherwise I think I would probably hate the word. I'd either be a patient or a sufferer, [both] of which I think are very loaded words really ... the connotation of being a victim is one that you know you try and keep away from really, that

you're being somehow … that you are a recipient of something, rather than actually doing something about it yourself … by the same token, personally myself, I absolutely hate the word patient … I absolutely loath the word. I carry a little card round with me, because I had my spleen removed as part of the treatment for Hodgkin's, I carry a little card. And on the front it says, 'I am a patient with no spleen'. And I would gladly tear it up and write my own. In fact one of these fine days I will, you know … it's something that absolutely I just hate. The 'patient' you know. And you know you're a patient … well I don't even like it when you're referring to somebody who's ill or in hospital, or you know going to see the doctor, or whatever. I still don't like the actual word itself. I think it has overtones of being a victim or disempowered.

(Kate: 31 yrs after diagnosis with ovarian cancer)

The concept of 'disempowerment' has been identified by both Katie and Kate and even after the length of time since their illnesses it clearly has intense meaning for them. For Kate it has even coloured her interpretation of how others are labelled and is perhaps indicative that 'negative labelling' during adolescence can have a life-long impact (Jacobs 1985). Lesley echoes these sentiments with the following comment:

[It] used to annoy me at the time, and still does now … when they say you know like 'oh she's battled with it', and you know, 'oh she's a trier, she'll come through'. And you think I'm damn sure every single person battles with it, and it's luck of the draw whether you come through it or not … You know it's nothing to do with personal … strength … I do find myself getting a bit … defensive about people who haven't managed to survive. It's not because they gave in … I wouldn't like people to be seen as victims of it.

(Lesley: 18 yrs after diagnosis with Hodgkin's lymphoma)

This quote is particularly significant as it places survivorship beyond the volitional and utterly rejects any consequent 'victim blaming' of those who do not survive. So not only do survivors not want to be seen as victims, they do not want those who did not survive to be interpreted as such either. Paul said that he identified himself as a cancer survivor and he too rejects the notion of 'victim' or 'sufferer':

I don't mind the word 'survivor', I hated you know the word sort of cancer victim or sufferer … ugh. Because it's not how it feels really but … I mean when I started this job – the job that I'm in now – you know you speak to people and you get to know them and, you know, and I would pick like long night shifts. I spoke to this woman at work and sort of like, 'Oh you poor thing, oh you … oh you were 18.' and she was starting to well up … I definitely did resist [victimhood], and I still do.

(Paul: 9 yrs after diagnosis with testicular cancer)

But for Quentin, 33 years after his diagnosis the notion of victimhood does not even enter his vocabulary or colour the much told story:

> I will tell the story if somebody gives me the chance as it were, the oppor-
> tunity … I'm still doing it now right at this very second, yes it's heroic …
> yes it's heroic … It's an important part of it, but in terms of this kind of
> almost false identity, or at least sort of knowing, you know reflects your
> identity. I know that the story can be presented in a kind of heroic or
> mock heroic light as it were. And I get a great deal out of presenting it in
> that way you know. And you know … and I survived and you know I
> enjoy that aspect of the story I suppose. You know, to myself as much as
> anything else I enjoy it you know. It's obviously an important part of my
> story, and has remained … and this has become more so I think over my
> life, the longer my life gets as it were the more worked out it gets, partic-
> ularly I think since my mid 30s.
>   (Quentin: 33 yrs after diagnosis with Hodgkin's lymphoma)

It seems significant that Quentin very consciously chooses to tell his story as an 'heroic' tale rejecting any element of vulnerability or victimhood, yet as he also says as a survivor of many years standing, the story has become increas-ingly important to him in that the way in which he presents it seems 'legendary', the result of many years of telling and retelling. Perhaps it is only after such a long period that the experience can be viewed with such equanimity.

I began my interview with Huxley, as with all the participants, by asking him to tell me what he had been diagnosed with and at what age. His response was to offer me a detailed account of the whole diagnostic process that, though it had occurred 18 years previously, was so detailed and apparently effortless to recall, it seemed that it could have happened very recently. Of course what Huxley was doing was, like Quentin did, to recount an often told and well-rehearsed account of his illness. As he said 'I've just told the story a thousand times, there's so many people interested, so many … they expect people to look like a victim or something.' There was nothing of the 'victim' about Huxley, an active sportsman who has worked as a gym instructor. He said the following about the way he told others of his past illness:

> The more you get to know people, the more people find out about the
> past. And sometimes I will blasély say at this particular period of my time I
> was … you know they might mention the word Christie's so 'oh well
> I've been there because I had cancer'. And that'll just be something that
> I've said to them, and then as soon as you say that people ask of your
> experience. So … I don't mind talking about it but I don't search to say
> 'look at me, I had cancer …' it's not like that. It's not that I'm embar-
> rassed about it, it just … it happened.
>   (Huxley: 18 yrs after diagnosis with acute lymphoblastic leukaemia)

For some survivors there was a need to engage in sponsored cancer-related activities, but for Elaine, her participation in the Race for Life to raise money, seemed at odds with her reluctance to discuss her illness with others:

> I do Race for Life every year ... I sort of wear a sign on my back saying you know I raced for life ... I find it reasonably hard to sort of talk about it, because it's obviously so personal to me ... my colleagues that I teach with at school, I think there's you know a couple of them who know, because it's sort of come up you know about the fact ... when we ... the whole school, you know well teacher did the Race for Life, so I was talking to sort of one of them about it, and sort of the reasons for doing it. It sort of comes up like that, but I certainly ... you know it's not something I've talked to many people about ... I don't know. It's very odd. It's just ... I don't know you know how I ... it just is quite hard to talk about it personally. You know how it affected me in that ... sort of just feel very self conscious about it I think, which you know I don't know that there's any reason why I should feel like that. I just do, if that makes any sense. I just ... I don't know ... I'm not a hugely sort of outgoing person anyway. But it's ... you know it's just ... I think it's just ... I find it quite difficult, because it's just talking about ... you know it's just about me, and sort of something that's obviously important to me.
>
> (Elaine: 5 yrs after diagnosis with Hodgkin's lymphoma)

In contrast Andrea had been interviewed by *Woman's Own* about her illness:

> I don't feel [like a victim] at all. No, I've never ... never felt that. In some ways it's given me an identity. [The interview] came about because I was invited to the 20 year celebration of the adult leukaemia unit being opened at Christies, because I was one of the first patients on the unit ... then *Woman's Own* picked that up from the Manchester Evening News. I was quite pleased really, because I'm always quite pleased to tell people my story, because I do think that whilst people are going ... are on with the treatment and they're going through it all, they never hear of any of the good side of things. It's all focused on treatment and people not making it, and it's all ... you know you tend to do hear about people that unfortunately haven't survived it, more than you do hear about people who have.
>
> (Andrea: 21 yrs after diagnosis acute myeloid leukaemia)

Andrea went on to say that in some ways her survivorship made her feel special and 'important' perhaps as a longer-term survivor like Quentin and Huxley, she is more able to accept the survivorship identity and incorporate it into her personal history and story even relishing its ability to distinguish her from the crowd. Elaine B relates a similar approach to telling her story:

There is no escape from it ... and once I open my mouth, I'm telling a whole story, it is a part of my identity now ... but it's positive. So I like to tell the story, because people ... everybody knows every ... somebody who's got cancer. And like I say, it's ... I'm a survivor so it's ... just because you have the big 'C', you can survive.

(Elaine B: 15 yrs after diagnosis with Hodgkin's lymphoma)

For Marc survivorship has become a primary component of his identity as his website shows. His many achievements such as being a Paralympic medal winner, his sponsored climb of the world's highest active volcano in aid of TCT and his work as a motivational speaker are arguably a direct result of his illness.

I kind of make a living out of telling my story, of which cancer is part of it. And so I do refer to it and talk about it a lot, yes.

(Marc: 21 yrs after diagnosis with osteosarcoma)

John too, in addition to his website, talks to groups about his cancer experience:

I've done a series of talks on the book and my experiences ... to cancer support groups, to nurses, to doctors, even did one to a number of pharmaceutical companies ... the women's institutes ... so anybody really who wants to hear an inspirational story ... even [after] all of these years down the line it's still very, very you know raw in the subconscious mind.

(John: 33 yrs after diagnosis with Hodgkin's lymphoma)

Similarly Ashley's cancer-related skin condition had resulted in him identifying himself primarily as a survivor and the rationale for him subsequently setting up a helpline for others with similar health problems:

I can argue that my whole being has been to a certain extent affected by a diagnosis at 17.

(Ashley: 37 yrs after diagnosis with CTCL)

One element that has been missing in these accounts is an explicit indication of whether there has been a particular and distinctive effect resulting from having been diagnosed in adolescence/young adulthood. It may be implicit in Ashley's last comment but Ben mentions it specifically and suggests that being diagnosed in adolescence/young adulthood inevitably shapes the forming of an emergent identity:

It's shaped how I am. You know it's quite a major ... especially only being 18 when I got it ... because it makes you mature a lot quicker as well ... yes I suppose it has changed my identity yes.

(Ben: 4 yrs after diagnosis with testicular cancer)

The examples in this chapter of taking on the identity of a cancer survivor in a very public way may not be how most survivors incorporate their illness history into their identity, but they are examples of how the illness has shaped lives in a very positive fashion and how survivorship identity can continue to be a defining characteristic for many years. However, distance from the event on its own is not enough to engender a sense of pride as we see from Linda:

> Most people don't know I've had it to be honest, you know like where I work. I never put it down on the form or anything like that. So it's something that just isn't talked about really. I just didn't want people singling me out and treating me differently, you know people tend to feel sorry for you and treat you differently. Like my mum treats me differently. I've got three sisters, and they're all healthy. But she does treat me ... she sort of you know, wraps me up in cotton wool a bit too much because she thinks I'm poorly all the time. And I'm not, I'm quite ... you know I'm fine like the rest of them really so ... it's probably stemmed from my mum actually.
>
> (Linda: 28 yrs after diagnosis with Hodgkin's lymphoma)

The crucial difference here may lie not just in Linda's resistance to being seen as a victim – which she shares with other participants – but in the fact that her mother, even 28 years on, still tends to treat her as though she was ill. So it seems that if the role of 'sufferer' and its association with vulnerability becomes embedded through the way in which others treat the survivor, this can have a far-reaching impact. Some of Scott's account resonates with Linda's but he provides an additional dimension of a contrasting combination of positivity and reluctance to be identified as a survivor. Scott moved to London from his home town in Scotland 5 years after his diagnosis and did not want anyone in his new life in the south to know of his illness. Rather than embracing the role of survivorship into his public identity, he deliberately chose to conceal this and said the following about why:

> So I made a point actually of – when I managed to get back to work after the transplant – of not telling people in work life what had happened to me ... and that was deliberately ... firstly I think there was an issue around probably getting a job in the first instance where you know if you'd been off ... if you hadn't worked for 6 months and you had some ongoing stuff going on then maybe companies wouldn't have looked at you so favourably – rightly or wrongly. So I got myself into this place where I didn't want people to know, because I felt it might affect my chances. And then the other side to that was I didn't want people to know because I didn't want them thinking ... well I didn't want people asking me how you feeling, how are you all the time. But also I just wanted to be treated like everyone else ... actually all through my ... career I've never mentioned it to anybody ... I would want people to say all the things that

they currently say which is you know this guy is a real expert in his field, you should speak to him about this, these are all the things that he's really great at. And I'd hate for them to be saying to someone oh and by the way did you know that you know he had cancer when he was younger.

(Scott: 18 yrs after diagnosis with ALL)

It is interesting that in contrast to Ashley, John and Marc – Scott, like Linda – very deliberately withheld his survivorship status fearing that this would construct him as a victim. He had already told me how much he had hated the sympathetic enquiries about his health that dominated his encounters with people after his diagnosis and did not want that replicated in his new working environment. He told me that he did not want anyone to think 'higher' of him because he was a cancer survivor and that it was important to him that his success in his chosen career, in the entertainment industry, was not dependent on any sympathy or special treatment he might have received as a cancer survivor. Yet this resistance to acknowledging his survivorship status seems to be at odds with the very positive way in which he felt the experience had shaped his outlook on life that is reminiscent of the testimonies in the last chapter:

Maybe 12/13 years post transplant, I started to look at the experience and what had happened to me as being incredibly positive. Because I think it had really set the tone for how I live my life in terms of keeping things in context in terms of their importance ... but I only actually noticed this in my early 30s ... The other element that I noticed was that I've got a very, very successful career, and I think part of the reason for that is because of ... I came out of the process wanting to you know, get the best out of every day and absolutely make the most of things. Hopefully I'd had a bit of that in me prior to being diagnosed anyway, but it certainly [gave] me an edge in a positive sense to drive on and to really try and lead the most fulfilled life that I could do. So I had a sense of perspective in terms of you know what was important, but also a sense of perspective in that you know this is your one shot at having a life, and you've absolutely got to grasp it. And through career, and relationships, and everything else, you know I really ... I think I've done exceptionally well. And I think what happened to me actually gave me a little bit of an edge and actually I think you know even potentially a nicer person. I really do, because you're able to deal with all the things that come your way every day. I think you're just ... you're better equipped ... to deal with life because there's not many things worse that can happen to you. And you know if something terrible like that happens to you in your teens, actually whilst it's an almighty blow at the time, it sets you up for ... things will continue to happen to you for the rest of your life, and there'll be good things and bad things. But the bad things will never be as bad as what's happened. You can almost park it and say that is really broadly speaking one of the worst things that's ever happened to me, and likely to happen to me. And as a result I'm better equipped than most people around me to actually push on in life and really maximise it.

(Scott: 18 yrs after diagnosis acute lymphatic leukaemia)

It is important in a volume of this sort that not only are the challenges understood, but also the ways in which the experience has shaped lives in a beneficial way, thus the next part of this chapter includes material that offers reflections on the enhanced sense of self resulting from pride in survivorship, this continues the theme of positive outcomes begun in the last chapter.

Positive outcomes

Julie's account of how her illness made her more assertive and confident, challenges any assumption that for a self confessed, overly cautious, worrier like Julie the advent of life-threatening illness would necessarily exacerbate an apparent inability to cope well with life. As we see from the following quotation the reverse seems to have been the case:

I'm [a] very, very cautious person, [it] stems from growing up being a constant worrier about things even as a child ... I mean I still bite my fingernails. And I used to hate being around people, and I used to get myself in a state about school and things like that. And I was a complete wreck really most of my time, especially during my teenage years and everything ... But when this happened [the illness] I know that my mum thought I would kind of just fall to pieces you know, because beforehand I'd had some bouts of depression, and all sorts of things. And you see, you'd think after all that kind of thing you wouldn't cope very well at all with having a diagnosis of cancer. But it's like brought me together kind of thing, it just seemed like just for once, you know I just got it together and just could get on with it. And in a strange sort of way – maybe it's me, I'm a hypochondriac or something – but it was like something to focus on. And you know how it's like often the fear of not knowing something is worse than knowing something ... The fear of the unknown. That's worse for me. So maybe ... I think I grew up with sort of ... all these fears of what might happen, and then when things do happen I'm you know ... I feel much more in control of things, as long as I have the facts and information ... I've been much more decisive and I've done so many more things I never thought I would do. Speaking up for your rights and questioning authority, and I just felt I was really a different person completely, because I wouldn't have done that beforehand ... I'm much more ... Yes, assertive I think. I am much more assertive than I was before. That's entirely the right word. I don't know if confident is the right word, but assertive is definitely.

(Julie: 15 yrs after diagnosis with Hodgkin's lymphoma)

So Julie's ability to face the worst and survive has given her a positive identity, she is a successful survivor. She is no longer someone to whom bad things happen – a victim – she is a person who can transcend misfortune. Paul B's account is strikingly similar as is Elaine B's:

> It made me grow up a lot ... I'm a lot more able to speak to people about sort of deeper issues ... I used to be very shy when I was at school, I was quite a shy person, but now I'm a lot more able to talk to people ... you'd have never seen me as a manager when I was at school. But since I've had this [the illness] I think maybe I'm a bit more laid back about things, and I'm a lot more easy going in terms of talking to people than I was.
>
> (Paul B: 11 yrs after diagnosis with non-Hodgkin's lymphoma)

> It's made me a lot more confident. I was very, very timid first ... before I used to go all coy and think oh no, I can't do that. And you just think no, sod it, I make a fool of myself or ... you know if you try these things ... I'm proud of myself, what I've done ... I've got through it, and there's a lot of friends that have ... you know I moan, and they've not got through it. And at the end of the day I'm here to tell the story. So you know I've fought it, and I'm proud of myself for fighting it.
>
> (Elaine B: 15 yrs after diagnosis with Hodgkin's lymphoma)

The concept of being proud was reflected on by Kirsty:

> Sometimes I think well actually yes, I did get over it. And I think there is something that you feel you know quite proud about yourself, even though you didn't, you know invent the chemotherapy or anything. But you did go through it. And I do think that definitely being a survivor is something that I am proud of. And you know that ... and I definitely do feel ... yes, I do feel like it's part of me now, because I suppose it's something I can't sort of erase from my past or anything like that.
>
> (Kirsty: 5 yrs after diagnosis with Hodgkin's lymphoma)

Kate told me that she had experienced depression in her late teens prior to her diagnosis and had had a very negative attitude towards life. However, in what may at first seem a surprising response to her cancer diagnosis, she feels that her current positive attitude can be attributed to the illness:

> I had depression when I was about 18 or 19 for quite a long time ... I had this sort of negative mental attitude to life, I've had to develop this positive mental attitude, where I don't worry about things or dwell on the past. But I try and look forward, because the future's the only thing you can actually change – and to try and be positive about it. So I make positive choices ... I've developed an attitude that says if something's horrible I'm going to change it if I can, and if I can't I'm going to try not to worry about it ... If I can do something I will ... I think it's come out of the

Hodgkin's ... because I think with depression it's actually quite difficult to change. Because if you are depressed you can't ... changing is actually the last thing you can do ... I just feel that that's actually a positive outcome from being so sick, really is that I have been able to think right you know, I'm going to take charge of my life, I'm going to make positive choices.

(Kate: 31 yrs after diagnosis with Hodgkin's lymphoma)

Again with Jamie, a person who acknowledges a tendency to depression, rather than exacerbating his depression the illness has given him an inner strength:

I've got depression ... but I don't know, I suppose really and truthfully it's made me a stronger person because I sit there and I think to myself well I've come through that and that's killing people all over the world, and I've come through it so it's made me feel like much a stronger person ... In a sense it's made me more positive, because when I sit there and think to myself it's like well some people die from that, but I've come through it and I'm fine, through the other side. So in a sense it's made me more positive. It affects me some days, but overall it's made me more positive.

(Jamie: 2 yrs after diagnosis with testicular cancer)

In addition to accounts of feeling greater confidence, stronger relationships were developed with family:

I suppose my family is quite a lot closer. I don't know if that's to do with growing up anyway. I think you accept your mum and dad as human beings a bit more as you grow out of your teens, but we're certainly a very close family.

(Jack: 9 yrs after diagnosis with Hodgkin's lymphoma)

And with friends:

I think that's been a good sort of thing as well because all my friends were in sixth form when they came to visit me. And we've really sort of stayed together. I mean I don't know if we would have done otherwise, but we really kept together as a group, and we're really close in a group you know. We've really ... I'm not sure how long that is – 10 years – almost 10 years on. But I think for them as well, I mean you know it was a big deal ... And it has been like that. So there's been positive aspects from the situation as well.

(Paul: 9 yrs after diagnosis with testicular cancer)

For Janet the positive impact had been to stop worrying about material things and events in the past she could not change:

Well I think certainly from a financial side of thing, I don't worry. I don't worry so much about money as perhaps … obviously sometimes if the bank's overdrawn I'm a bit concerned, but you know I don't get sort of really … don't worry about material things. And I don't know, I think I have a very positive outlook on things – always have had. And people say that to me, because you know I just … I'm very … I suppose you know the saying no point crying over spilled milk, I don't get worried about things that have happened, there's no point, it's happened. And I do feel I have a positive outlook on things really.

(Janet: 27 yrs after diagnosis with Hodgkin's lymphoma)

This positive attitude is echoed by Gillian:

Positive for me was … after it … I got married, I started a new life as it were … and then started a family … every time there's a milestone … within the family like … gosh I mean when my granddaughter was born I was just so emotional because … I just never thought I would see her. But that's the positive side; you know every step that goes on is … it did change the way … I grew up I guess although I was 20, but I grew up. I think I missed out kind of a stage, because … you're suddenly … an adult, face things that most of your own age group aren't facing. And so you do grow up I think that bit older. But yes, it's … it is a positive thing. It's something that you've had in your life, you've got through it, and you feel well if I can get through that I can get through other things … The whole thing is positive … I sort of think well you know in a way yes, I'm quite special to have had it … you sort of think well you know I am, I'm special, I've done this, I've had this, got through it, beaten that. My body has beaten it … but yes. I'm not saying I'd want to go through it again.

(Gillian: 34 yrs after diagnosis with Hodgkin's lymphoma)

Debbie echoed Bob's (see Chapter 2) commitment to caring for his patients, she too had been traumatised by the way in which her diagnosis was originally given and could empathise with the need for a sympathetic approach. Her account is also similar to John's approach to his patients:

Yes, definitely how I react to patients, very much so. And obviously where I teach [dental school] … we're linked to the radiotherapy unit, so we have people coming you know, pre-radiotherapy and that sort of thing. And again, sometimes I do tell them that I've had it myself, because again just that reassurance to people. But also so that they know you do actually understand. You know, that doctor that gave me my original diagnosis would probably say to you of course I understand how you're feeling. There's no way he could have done, because he wouldn't have talked to me like that. So … and I do have a reputation – both at the practice and at the hospital – for being particularly caring. I think it's made me very

warm, definitely. I've sat in with oral surgeons that have had to tell someone they're going to have their tongue removed for oral cancer and that
sort of thing. And again, I sit there and think I wish I'd had someone like
you to talk to me. That was fantastic. I mean that's devastating news ...
worse than mine was. And to be spoken to in such a lovely way just makes
me think about it again you know ... it never, ever leaves you – or it's
never, ever left me. And I am just incredibly grateful to be here. I really,
really am ... I don't ever wish it hadn't happened, because it's really made
me who I am ... I think I'm a much, much better person for it.

(Debbie: 22 yrs after diagnosis with Hodgkin's lymphoma)

We have already established that survivorship had become integral to Marc's
identity, in a way made much more public than for many survivors. From his
account, which follows, it seems that his sporting prowess, while pre-dating
his illness, was enhanced by the experience rather than – as might have been
anticipated – diminished by it:

I was a reasonably good sportsperson before this happened, but I was
pretty lazy ... I would just rely on the small amount of talent I had to get
by, but wouldn't practice or train or anything. And the frame of mind
that I gained encouraged me to train better, and then once I started doing
that I actually realised that I could achieve quite a lot doing that. I was
swimming quicker with one leg than before when I had two. And I used
to be a county swimmer. So it made me realise actually if I did apply
myself physically then I could achieve a lot, lot more. And as I've grown
up I suppose I've become more aware of the kind of power of that kind of
positive attitude if you want to call it – an overused phrase but that kind
of ... the frame of mind that if you have a frame of mind you can achieve
a lot of things. I do a lot of climbing now, where at every single step your
body is telling you to turn around and go back down because it's so
fatiguing. But I know that most of it is in your mind. And I think that's ...
it's a mental legacy really, but it drives the physical legacy, if that makes
sense ... I'm very, very philosophical about things, and if that door closes
then there's other doors that open. In actual fact I lost a leg but I gained
so much more. If you had to sum up my whole attitude about it, that
would be it – I lost my leg but I gained a respect for life.

(Marc: 21 yrs after diagnosis with osteosarcoma)

Ashley too had adopted a very public profile as a direct result of an ongoing
interconnectedness with his own cancer experience, this had resulted in what
he perceived as a very positive outcome, not only for himself but for others
undergoing similar illnesses:

[It's] 15-odd years since I made a documentary for the BBC called
'Scratching the Surface' ... I did do a lot of research prior to the making

of that documentary. And following that up has enabled me to hopefully put myself in a position where I can be of assistance to people, and there is a lot of pain out there. So that's what I do on a daily basis, and feel incredibly privileged that I can put my head on the pillow at the end of each day and feel as if I've made a positive difference in someone's life, which not everybody can say, but it's a brilliant thing to do when you're in that position ... The positive effects of living with this ... is like I've had over the 37-odd years has had a very positive effect in some ways. And there are choices that I've made that have been brilliant ... I have tried to pack so much into my life, because you know there was every chance that I wouldn't have the three score years and 10 that most people expect, because of a diagnosis so young.

(Ashley: 37 yrs after diagnosis with CTCL)

Finally, Greg who without having constructed his life around campaigning, educating others or achieving survivor-related goals made the following comment:

You know it's all positive. You can see life in a more positive way. Not that I ever looked, looked at it in a negative way but I mean I just think everything about it is fantastic.

(Greg: 19 yrs after diagnosis with osteosarcoma)

There were many other comments that denote positive effects and some of them are implicit in quotes used elsewhere in this volume. For example, the quotes at the end of Chapter 5 largely represent an enhanced appreciation of life. But here I have tried to offer a range of viewpoints that both reinforce and complement one another through a selection from survivors of both genders and different time spans who found positivity in different ways.

Summary

The notion of the embeddedness of identity as a survivor is strong in the earlier accounts. However long the period since diagnosis, that identity continues to be integral – it may change and the story may become 'heroic' as told and retold over decades as we saw with Quentin and Huxley – but it continues to shape how survivors perceive themselves. It may also be the case that the length of time that has elapsed since the illness is a contributory factor in the experience being viewed in a positive light. It is perhaps not coincidental that so many of the quotations under the 'Positive outcomes' heading are from longer-term survivors; yet we also see that those much closer to the illness, like Kirsty and Jamie, can interpret the experience as having had a positive legacy.

It is interesting that while identity emerged as being significant, so many of the participants followed swiftly and emphatically with a qualification that they would hate to be perceived as vulnerable or as being 'victims' or 'sufferers'. They abhorred any element of 'pity' or special pleading that might be evoked and one even eschewed the label of 'patient'. Many regarded the illness with which they had been diagnosed as pivotal to their subsequent successful development, this was a source of pride and, in many cases, their survivorship identity was a public, continuing and significant feature of their lives. However, it was important that it was not assumed that allowances had been made for them as a result of their illness.

In contrast to those who 'went public' there were also accounts from survivors who felt uncomfortable at disclosing their status as survivors, though these were in the minority. Because of the nature of the research and the size of the sample I can offer no generalisation of why this might have been the case apart from observing that both Linda and Scott feared being treated as vulnerable or invalids and in Linda's case this appears to be connected to her mother's tendency to 'wrap her in cotton wool' and Scott worked in the competitive environment of the entertainment industry. However it is also the case that even some participants like Dan and Thomas who had been identified publicly as survivors wished to move on from what they perceived to be a defining identity and be known for their other achievements. The resistance to being identified primarily as a survivor may be supportive of Jacob's (1985) theory of the tendency to reacting badly to being labelled, but there is evidence in many of the accounts that rather than becoming 'stuck' in their identity at the point of diagnosis, if the right sort of support and opportunities are available, survivors can transcend a negative label.

The pride with which they regarded their survivorship seems in many cases to have resulted in an enhanced sense of identity and self worth. This raises the issue of whether identity for these survivors carries with it a distinct quality because they were diagnosed during adolescence and young adulthood when other identities may be fragile and incomplete (Grinyer 2002a). There are some implicit indications that this is the case as it seems that having survived life-threatening illness at this transitional stage has changed the course of lives in a way that might not be the case with much younger or older people.

In addition to the implicit suggestions that this is the case, there are also some more explicit indications. For example, both Ben and Scott say that having the illness in their teens, at that particular stage of life, shaped who they were and how they subsequently viewed and lived their lives. Gillian notes the sudden maturity into adulthood having missed out a life stage. To have undergone such an experience at this age sets the survivors apart from their peers, this will not only have had an impact on life plans, as we see in the next chapter, it will also have had an effect on what Marc calls the 'mental legacy' at a crucial moment in the life trajectory.

The effect of being set apart from peers is what may make identity as a survivor of cancer in adolescence/young adulthood 'special'; indeed some participants said that it made them feel 'special'; such an unexpected life event may carry with it an enhanced significance and meaning. Thus, I would argue that from the data presented here there is more evidence of Frank's (2002) 'obligation of the cured' than what McKenzie and Crouch (2004) describe as a situation in which 'their very identities – indelibly inscribed by the cancer experience – are pushed to the margins of the social fabric in which selfhood is embedded' (2004: 143).

Nevertheless, it seems crucial to the nature of survivorship identity that it precludes any suggestion of vulnerability and is instead regarded by self and others as a matter of pride. There are accounts here of survivors who have constructed their lives around their survivorship identity in very public ways while others carry their identity with them with pride but privately. Yet in both cases it seems that the survivor identity is internalised and central for many years.

Key Points

Identity

* The identity of 'survivor' can become central
* This identity can last for many decades
* The mantle of survivorship may become more meaningful as time passes
* There is complete rejection of being perceived as a 'victim' or 'sufferer' or as being vulnerable
* Survivorship can bring strength and assurance to those who had previously felt vulnerable

Positive outcomes reported

* Improved relationships with family and friends
* Greater empathy with others who are ill
* Greater confidence
* A sense of purpose and focus

---

7 The effect on life plans and the long-term financial impact

The life stage at which young adults have been diagnosed with cancer is a crucial point on the life trajectory when key decisions are being made and opportunities seized – and lost – thus the ramifications of disruption can have far-reaching consequences (Grinyer 2002a, 2007). However, Levitt and Eshelman (2008) say that there has been little thus far that could provide evidence that describes the impact on educational achievements, problems in the workplace, the effect on employment status and access to financial services such as insurance and mortgages. Nevertheless, these authors cite American studies that suggest that there is resulting discrimination in the workplace and financial sector.

Advances in cancer treatments and changing attitudes have, according to Hoffmann (2007), led to an expansion of the legal rights of cancer survivors in the workplace. However, she argues that despite there being fewer blatant barriers to opportunities many survivors still attribute vocational problems to their cancer. Fobair (2007) identifies some of the possible barriers to successful employment such as: having a reduced capacity for strenuous work, greater fatigue, problems communicating comfortably with an employer and difficulty in gaining promotion. If such harmful impacts are being experienced in the wider cancer survivor population, the effect on those at the start of careers may be exacerbated.

Soliman and Agresta (2008) suggest that this age group is particularly vulnerable to the financial effects of a cancer diagnosis. They find it difficult to obtain insurance as they are considered high-risk and in interviews with 227 survivors of childhood cancer 11 percent reported some form of employment-related discrimination. Again this study is based on childhood cancer rather than adolescent and young adult cancer and this chapter seeks to contribute to knowledge of this age group in these areas.

As Langeveld and Arbuckle (2008: 153) point out, it can be difficult for the young survivor to resume their studies or work after such a life-changing experience and this effect will be compounded by the gap in their education or employment record. My research enables us to chart the longer-term effects of these issues and of other broader life plans that may have been changed, damaged or in some cases enhanced, by the illness.

We begin with Maz whose working life seems to have been dealt a severe blow by his illness:

> I want just to be back on my track, which I do miss at the moment. I want to go back where I used to [be] working. I'm not asking so much but I want to do a decent job. I want to stand up on my foot, nobody ... to accuse me or abuse me, like I'm different walking and stuff like that. But sometimes they just given me help because I can't walk really well. That's the thing I don't want to ... I'm not ... accepting this stuff you see and this it gives me [a] headache sometimes, that's why I just ... upset myself you see ...
>
> (Maz: 4 yrs after diagnosis with Ewing's sarcoma)

It is clear that Maz feels he is judged and discriminated against because he no longer has the physical stamina to carry out the manual work he once did. A very similar response was given by Majad who also said he could not do any lifting and this had affected his ability to return to work:

> I can't work. You know like in a way, if I was working I wouldn't work because I couldn't pick up anything heavy ... it has made my life a bit, you know down. You know like knowing I've got cancer.
>
> (Majad: 7 yrs after diagnosis with testicular cancer)

His wife Rizwana told me the following while Majad was moving his car. The far-reaching changes the testicular cancer had brought, not only to his ability to work but to every aspect of his life, are apparent:

> He was doing two jobs. He was doing really well for himself. Honestly he was working, he had you know ... he had his car, you know he had like all his friends around him, his family, he had me you know ... I think he's his parents' favourite. So whatever he wants they give it him ... and now he hardly even like goes to see his parents, because it's like ... when he sees them after a long time they like ask him, oh how's your cancer going, you know do you go for your check-ups, and it's all back again ... he doesn't really go anywhere, because he's always like ... oh he's like ... oh he's always got this thing oh I'm going to die one day and I want to make the most of my kids. So he's always at home with me. Even if I say let's go to the cinema, no I don't want to go because it's that you know 'I don't want to go out'. He's tried so many times like to get a job, to go to work. And then he just [can't] ... like lifting heavy things or driving and stuff that ... because he loves driving but when he's driving for too long he's like oh I'm tired now.
>
> (Rizwana: Majad's wife)

The emotional effect on Maz of being unable to work and the far-reaching impact on Majad's life are evident 7 years after his diagnosis. However, Meg spoke to me considerably longer after her illness, her whole working life had been affected by the physical legacy of her lymphoma and she had eventually been forced to take early retirement in her early 40s because of the neuropathy in her arm:

> I had neuropathy in my right shoulder, so it was affecting my right arm. I mean I know I'm left handed, the job I was doing kind of needed both arms ... it had started to affect my shoulder a year or so down the line. You know just gradually, but nothing too much. And I thought I was being like kind of – how can I say – a bit clumsy at first. And I realised ... and then I started getting pains, and you know and I'd said to them at the hospital ... and they said 'oh you know'. And then I said I had pains again, and then they put me into the hospital, into the neurology department and it was diagnosed as neuropathy ... because they'd burnt all the nerves in my right shoulder.
>
> (Meg: 38 yrs after diagnosis with Hodgkin's lymphoma)

Maz, Majad and Meg had all worked in occupations that required some physical stamina and strength and had clearly found a return to work too challenging despite their expressed desire to resume their working lives. However, for Kristin, who it first appeared did not appear have any concrete ambitions or plans, and who had almost willingly embraced the sick role (Parsons 1951), his illness had allowed and even encouraged him to opt out of taking an active and participative role:

> I'm getting free money so I might wait until that finishes [to look for work]. My muscles were proper weak when I came out, you know after my last treatments. But once they start strengthening up I might lose my free money sort of thing, so I'll have to start working. And I wouldn't mind going back to where I left off, if I'm allowed.
>
> (Kristin: 4 yrs after diagnosis with testicular cancer)

However, Kristin then talked about the things his illness would prevent him from doing in the longer-term:

> I am interested in electronics, and piping sort of stuff. Like being a plumber. So I wouldn't mind actually getting a course on to that ... Some jobs I won't be able to do ... Like plenty of walking about. Like one of the jobs before I had all this treatment, well it was just like standing all day, and making boxes. It's that sort of thing I won't be able to do ... I can't be on my feet for too long. But ... word from the doctor is that everything won't go back to where it was, of my strength and feeling. Like it went down, but it's only going up so far.
>
> (Kristin: 4 yrs after diagnosis with testicular cancer)

So again we see that for a young man whose options appear to be limited to manual labour the limitation of employment opportunities is far-reaching. While Kristin had already told me that his life was not so different than it had been previously as he was and had always been an avid player of computer games in his bedroom, he did acknowledge that life might be different had he not had the illness, his tendency to isolate himself socially having been exacerbated by the cancer:

> I'd probably be out and about more than actually kicking around at home. But I had ... I had a better life then ... Yes, because I'd have met a lot more people. Like now, just one mate ... well two mates and that's it.
> (Kristin: 4 yrs after diagnosis with testicular cancer)

Jamie was unemployed when I interviewed him, but had in fact just left a job at the time of his diagnosis. He had eventually taken up employment again 6 months after his treatment but his job had not lasted as he had subsequently experienced depression:

> I'd just left a job because ... before I got diagnosed I was just constantly getting pains, so I was at the doctor's all the time. And there was one day when it just really, really got on top of me and I couldn't walk. So I just ... I had to leave my job. So I was lucky in a sense that I could recover fully from my operation. So I was actually unemployed when it was diagnosed but ... I actually got depression last year, so it sort of like I had to leave that job because it was a case of just talking it through with the boss, it's like well just go get your head sorted out and then come back ... come back to work when you've sorted yourself out. Just sort of like getting that under control and then getting a job, and then from there just being a normal person. Just living every day like everybody else does. Just go to work, come home, have your fun and then go to work next day.
> (Jamie: 2 yrs after diagnosis with testicular cancer)

Jamie's wish to be 'just like a normal person' seems to be connected in his perception to working and then having 'permission' to have fun earned through having been at work, but for Julie, who had also had to relinquish her job when diagnosed, the effect had been that her focus had turned towards home and family rather than combining family commitments and paid employment:

> I think if I hadn't of had that Hodgkin's I think my decisions would have been different. I think I would have definitely ... maybe gone back to work and been a bit more of a working mum, and instead of just wanting to sort of hold on to everything and be at home. It's turned me into a homing person.
> (Julie: 15 yrs after diagnosis with Hodgkin's lymphoma)

For Ben it was the stress related to his job that meant he had to seek alternative employment and it is apparent that it is his belief that to be put under stress may cause a relapse or exacerbate his cancer:

> I used to manage retail outlets and it was very, you know stressful. You know targets and, you know … you know just hassle all the time. But I work now for a distribution centre … it's a lot less stressful, you know you do your own job and that's it. It's as simple as that really … in a way it's bad … you're just a number. You know whereas before I was somebody who had responsibility and, you know, had other people to sort out what they were doing, whereas now I've got no stress at all with work. So that's one good thing, I've got 40 hours a week and I've no stress. I just go do my job and then come home. And as soon as I walk out of that job I don't think about … I've read in places, you know stress making cancer worse and I think it did, like make it worse … I do think about that quite a bit.
>
> (Ben: 4 yrs after diagnosis with testicular cancer)

The accounts thus far could all be interpreted as negative in their tone. However in Quentin's case, while he had had to take a year out of university to recover from his treatment for Hodgkin's lymphoma, rather than having a detrimental impact on his educational trajectory he used the time to immerse himself in political ideology through extensive reading:

> I did politics, history and law in my first year, and by the end of the first year I decided I wanted to do politics, so I became sort of radicalised, left-wing by the end of the first year. I probably considered myself in some sense a Marxist by the end of the first year, but in that reading in the year I had out, I formed a definite idea of what I … I thought I knew what I thought by the time I got to university … And so the first thing I did when I got back [was to join] the International Socialists … so I immediately went into student/revolutionary politics, as soon as I got back … and I was a bit of a phenomenon really, even if I do say so myself … one of the things I did, even as an undergraduate [was] running Capital readers groups … unlike most people, and probably with some justification [I felt] that I understood it … so I was a bit of a phenomenon in that sense I suppose.
>
> (Quentin: 33 yrs after diagnosis with Hodgkin's lymphoma)

Paul had also taken a year out after his diagnosis and while he resumed his studies, after his enforced and resented interruption, he was uncertain about the extent to which his current profession in mental health has been shaped by his illness experience:

> I was going to university when it first … I did go back [but] I took a year [out], because I was in the first year so I basically I just … I quit first year,

and you know redid the first year after I'd finished. There was no sense that I wasn't going to do that. I mean I was just ... you know determined and kind of you know, how dare this thing sort of interrupt my life. I work in mental health ... as a support worker, I'm a warden and I enjoy that job a lot. And I'm not sure ... it's hard to say but I mean I'm not sure, I mean I'm not sure I wouldn't have done that anyway ... It's a question I've asked myself as well. Sort of like you know [a] number of times sort of, 'how did I get into this?' I guess ... it does have its own sort of mental health sort of part to it, going through cancer.

(Paul: 9 yrs after diagnosis with testicular cancer)

Elaine too had had her education disrupted and had been forced to take time out. While she went back to her course and qualified, a crucial meeting with the man she was to marry would not have occurred without the illness. The fact that this chance meeting that was to change her life would not have happened without the cancer was not lost on her:

When I was diagnosed I'd just started a ... PGCE course, and I sort of decided that because of the way I was I didn't want to carry it on that year, and I put it off for a year. And actually sort of I think my life has changed, and sort followed a different path, because I put the PGCE off course for a year, that I think well actually if I hadn't have had cancer you know my life could have been quite different ... But that I mean that sounds silly but it's like you know, I ended up living with my best friend and I met my partner through her and ... I feel like where I am now would have been completely different if I hadn't had it.

(Elaine: 5 yrs after diagnosis with Hodgkin's lymphoma)

Kelly too had taken a PGCE and qualified as a teacher, but though she had succeeded in completing her course she felt that the way she had been treated because of her illness was undermining when she tried to get a job:

I had to apply for my PGC year, and then I had to apply for it again for my NQT year, and both times I've been rung up by occupational health trying to find out whether I'm actually fit for the job ... I actually find it quite offensive that they have asked me that after 6 years, just because I've been truthful on my form. I don't mind you know somebody ringing up and being nice about it, but it's the sort of the implication that you've had it so you can't possibly be well enough to do a job ... the way that they approached it wasn't in a 'how can we help you?' way, it was in a 'are you right for the job then?'.

(Kelly: 7 yrs after diagnosis with non-Hodgkin's lymphoma)

Kelly may have been delayed by her illness in getting to university but she was able to complete her studies. However, in contrast, for Thomas the disruption to his university career did not have such a satisfactory outcome:

Well, no I didn't get back to physical uni ... I managed to get a recognition of the work that I'd done, a sort of one year diploma they called it. And so I tried to continue doing a degree ... I was doing a degree at Bristol Uni in Theology and Religious Studies and I tried to continue that when I was well enough with the Open University, with a Philosophy course, because the two ... go quite nicely, but unfortunately I was ill again.

(Thomas: 13 yrs after diagnosis with a brain tumour)

While Thomas's inability to return to his studies had clearly impacted on his education, the accompanying social effect had also been detrimental; he spoke about the social isolation it had caused and the resulting effect on the chances of meeting a girlfriend:

I mean I haven't had a relationship with a girl for God knows how many years. And that makes me very sad really, because when you're a teenager of course, you know diagnosed at 17, that's the point that you really begin to interact with the other sex. And you make relationships and so on, and I never had the opportunity as such, and I've never really been at school in a positive ... in a long sense ... or a university, or work. So I've never had a chance to develop those things. And you know that's sad for me at ... I feel at 30 that that should be the thing.

(Thomas: 13 yrs after diagnosis with a brain tumour)

Thomas's physical limitations also affected his social life in other ways:

It's unfortunate because part of the problem with the seizures is that I can become sort of hypersensitive to noise. And it really sort of, I don't know, freaks me out for want of a better term. But I ... sometimes [have to] actually remove myself ... actually in the wider sense it's sort of like sensory input – I can't deal with it sometimes, when I've been particularly bad in the past with seizures ... and also I can't drive ... so I mean ... I can't do things like go out. I mean thinking back to ... well uni and so on, people obviously walk out to the pub. Yes, I could get a taxi to the pub, because I couldn't walk, but I would have missed all the chat ... I do feel that my illness has prevented me from having a really good friend, you know like a best mate who you would perhaps talk to and so on.

(Thomas: 13 yrs after diagnosis with a brain tumour)

Thomas articulates powerfully the age specific impact of the illness and its potential for long-term disruption to lives not yet established in terms of education, career or relationships. We can see that if the life trajectory is interrupted at this stage the impact may be felt for years. However, most survivors had established relationships – some of them were even attributed indirectly to the illness. Richard said he would not have met his wife had he not been trying to recover his fitness by attending a particular sporting event. Like Elaine,

Andrea said that she felt that she had married her first husband partly as a result of having been ill although in her case this was a marriage that had not been lasting. Indeed it was her enforced need to relinquish her career as an acrobatic dancer, and her resulting lack of confidence and disappointment, that appears to have led her to marriage:

I think I did, because I met him ... I met him obviously after I'd been ill. But I was only ... it was only about a year after I'd been ill I met him. And because I was finding it such a hard time to get over the illness, not ... I wouldn't say over the illness, but getting back to any sort of a normal life. You know, a lot of my friends that I knew before I'd been ill had gone their own way, and you know I'd sort of been in hospital for a good 6 months more or less you know. And I didn't have ... there [weren't] a lot of friends that I had that were left around. And I found it hard to get out and meet people because my confidence wasn't there. It took me a long time to build my confidence back up. And I remember wishing at times that I hadn't got through it. That was ... it was a bad time getting over it. I tried to decide what to do with my life, because having the leukaemia meant that I couldn't carry on ... because I was a dancer. I was an acrobatic dancer. And I'd gone to work as a Blue Coat at Pontins, and that was just before I was diagnosed with leukaemia. And all through my treatment I was thinking I'm going to get back to it, I'm going to go back to it. But then obviously after the treatment I just tried my best to get back and do the dancing and the acrobatics, but I just was so disheartened, because I had no energy whatsoever. I couldn't get through it. And because I didn't have any support from anybody else, because all my friends ... had gone off, and it was a very hard time sort of accepting that really I wasn't going to carry on with being an entertainer like I'd dreamt of for a long, long time. It changed my life then. And I think that's for the years, like I say, of me blaming the leukaemia, that's what I blamed it on mostly you know. Where I would be now, doing something I'd always dreamt of doing. But then I decided to go to college. I'd tried one or two jobs, but because I was still quite weak and got tired very, very easily, I couldn't really stick at anything that I really enjoyed. I did hotel reception, which I really enjoyed, but the hours just ... I couldn't hack the hours. So then I decided to go back to college, and I chose to do beauty therapy, which I really enjoyed. But even going through college I found hard, because I was still raw from it really. And my confidence wasn't a 100 per cent at all.

(Andrea: 21 yrs after diagnosis with acute myeloid leukaemia)

However, at the time of the interview Andrea had set-up her own business and felt, that despite her disappointment at her dancing career being terminated and her various failed attempts at other career options, she had nevertheless found an occupation that satisfied her and she had also remarried.

Thus 21 years after her diagnosis she was able to take a longer-term perspective, but if I had interviewed her 10 years earlier the depiction of her life and the damage caused by the illness might have been related in a very different way.

Elaine B had been diagnosed with two different cancers 2 years apart and told me that her career as a professional ice skater had been affected seriously as a result:

> Yes, at the height of my career in *Disney on Ice*. So I even was abroad skating. And I had to give up the skating. And I didn't have a house or anything. My life was touring the world with a skating company ... [the company] kept my career on hold for a year. I was on chemotherapy, and then radiotherapy, and then obviously I had to get my stamina back up, and for a year I was out. And I went back after a year, with the doctor's signature. And they kept my place open for me ... I skated, and I was in New York, and I collapsed on the ice ... I knew it was back. So I went to the doctor's in New York, and I asked for an x-ray. And I could see a shadow. And then I flew home the next day. And they took ... they gave me keyhole surgery on this tumour, and that unfortunately ... that was the start of my second one. That was cancer ... Well strangely enough they still said there's always a place for me. So I was honoured. So the second time I was off again. Although they didn't keep my place ... once I was back I got in touch with Disney and after ... about a year later, and went skating, and everything was fine. Until I came home on vacation, went to the doctor's, just for normal pills and things, and that's when I had the lump in my stomach and I was [pregnant]
> (Elaine B: 15 yrs after first diagnosis with Hodgkin's lymphoma)

The impact of the unexpected pregnancy is discussed fully in the next chapter, and is yet another example of how Elaine B's life plans were dramatically altered as a result of the illness, in this case because she had assumed the treatment had left her infertile and had taken no precautions against becoming pregnant. Paradoxically, in the end it was the pregnancy not the cancer which terminated her ice skating career, though from her account we can se how disrupted her life and career had been as a result of her illness. Similarly, Kirsty was training as a dance teacher when she was diagnosed and at first was determined that her activities would not be curtailed. While she is uncertain that ultimately her career path was changed by her illness, she does acknowledge the impact:

> I probably shouldn't have done ... [but] just after I'd had my biopsy actually in my neck and my bone marrow, I was dancing a week and a half later. And I was absolutely determined that I was going to do it. And everyone said 'no'. And I know I should have listened to them, but it didn't do me any harm in the end. But I felt it was something I'd started.

Because I'd trained for like God knows how long to do this exam and it just … you know I thought oh God you know, the timing is just impeccable [ironic]. And I did my dancing exam and things like that. So it didn't stop me at first … [but the] biopsies and exploratory sort of surgeries and things like that that knocked me for six … I've actually ceased to teach dancing now … I did try and teach dancing a couple of nights a week because it was something that I'd done since I was tiny, and I'd loved it. And I wanted to keep sort of you know, a hand in somewhere. But getting back from London, it was just too tiring. And again my specialist wasn't quite happy about me overexerting myself and stressing myself out about getting home for you know a couple of evenings a week just to teach dancing. So it was something I decided okay fine, I will kind of you know, get on with my proper job now. And so I don't do that anymore, which is a shame … my specialist was saying you know you've got to take it easy, minimal stress, and you know don't you know exhaust yourself, don't get too tired. And I think because I'd just started working full time in London … because I mean although I was teaching dancing before, it was never full time … But I don't know, it's something I might have just had to stop anyway, whether I'd been ill or not. But that's one of the things I think, you know you don't really know what normal is after you've been ill because you can't sort of … there's nothing to compare it to. But I would say yes, it probably did play quite a big factor in it, yes.

(Kirsty: 5 yrs after diagnosis with Hodgkin's lymphoma)

Scott had almost made the grade as a professional footballer at the time of his diagnosis and his career path had taken a very different direction as a result:

I was a very fit and strong guy. I was almost a professional footballer, and I'd still been playing football right up to the point I was diagnosed. And I stayed in remission for about 18 months after that, and then sadly I relapsed.

(Scott: 18 yrs after diagnosis with ALL)

Scott has since established a successful career in the entertainment industry, but was clearly devastated at the time when his chances of being a professional footballer were dashed and he spoke with nostalgia over what might have been. Paul B was also training for a profession that required physical stamina and he relates the loss of confidence he felt to his illness:

I did a degree in sports science. And I think because I went back to university after the treatment, obviously I was extremely unfit. And I think that … in terms of the degree itself, it made me sort of take a back [seat] … I was always the one that sort of stuck back. And I think people maybe looked at me and [wondered] 'why's he standing back? So I think yes, maybe my confidence in the degree did get hindered ... I could have done a lot better with the degree itself. Yes, that's one thing I think it really did affect. And I might have taken sports science further that way. But I'd got so fed up of getting sort of put back with the education.

(Paul B: 11 yrs after diagnosis with non-Hodgkin's lymphoma)

While it may be understandable that for a manual worker, athlete, dancer or professional ice skater a cancer diagnosis would almost inevitably threaten their career, for a nurse it is perhaps less likely to have a lasting detrimental impact. Indeed some of the participants took up medical training as a result of their diagnosis. However, for Gillian her dream of qualifying as a children's nurse ended with her diagnosis:

The matron at the time – and I have to say she was a diabetic so she was obviously taking time off for clinics – she actually said to me ... 'you know you've had this, you're going to ... end up having to take time off for clinics, you're probably going to have more illnesses', she said 'I'm not prepared to keep you on, and I'm not letting you on a ward' ... she was going to put me in the milk room doing up the feeds and then do my finals and then I was out. In fact she was letting me do SEN, not SRN and children's. I could do my SEN and then I was out. And that wasn't what I wanted to do ... It was very difficult to get a job because you had to give your immediate medical history and that. It was impossible to get a job ... I did go back to work once both children were a little bit older. I just took a cleaning job at a weekend, which is when my husband could have the children. It was milking, it was a cheese dairy, it's you know not quite what it sounds, but ... and then I went on to work in the office, and I've worked for the same boss now for 22 years.

(Gillian: 34 yrs after diagnosis with Hodgkin's lymphoma)

While there may now be legislation to prevent the discrimination that Gillian experienced after her diagnosis, there are nevertheless long-term survivors who are still living with this type of impact on their careers. In a similar vein, Richard told me that he had lost out on a job after his diagnosis and that his career had been profoundly affected:

I was going to go from school into college, and so that got stopped. And I then started to study in a different direction, because the only job I could get was as a trainee accountant. And when I was in hospital they gave the job to somebody else ... And so I came out of hospital without a job, and no prospects of being able to go to university or college. And I was very lucky, I found myself in a situation where I could get another job with another organisation where they were more prepared to see me through the illness. And I stayed there for, you know, about 6 years as I went through that. But it was probably never going to be the career that I really wanted, but I just had to do it.

(Richard: 36 yrs after diagnosis with aggressive fibro sarcoma)

Richard told me that originally he had wanted to study art but that at no time since his diagnosis had he been able to return to his early ambition. Lisa told me a similar story about having graduated from university and begun a career in Human Resources (HR) but the illness had changed both her physical ability to manage the demands and her attitude to what was important:

I don't work – I've chosen not to work now. I have changed mentally. I think before I had the cancer I was … yes on the verge of my career really – at the beginning of it. I had gone to university, it was my first proper job as such, I was putting all my energies into my career. Well my perspective is very different from that now … I'd done my degree in human resources and then had a job in HR. And my company were very good. They obviously had long-term sick leave, and [I] went back, and they were very good at … I did part time for a long time. And I never actually went back full time. I only ever did four days a week. And then my focus then was the children aspect, whether we'd adopt, or egg donation, or whatever. And then after I had my first child I went back two days a week. And then since my second I've decided not to go back at [all] … it's completely related to being ill … [it] absolutely changed my priorities.

(Lisa: 9 yrs after diagnosis with non-Hodgkin's lymphoma)

In contrast, Jack's work had been shaped directly by his illness and at the time I interviewed him he was writing a play based on his experience of cancer:

Interestingly enough I'm writing a play at the moment for radio and it's … about a boy who's dying, and he's 15 … and he gets a wish … He wishes to sleep with a woman, because he's never slept with a woman. That's what sets him on this kind of adventure. I rang up the chap at the hospital to speak to him about, you know doing research, because of the pre-cancer involved, and he said a lot of people have biographical pain when they're in hospital because they've written their biographies now in their heads, and this wasn't supposed to happen you know. It shakes up everything and you have to re-write all your life. I suppose that's what happens. It just shakes you up, and it shakes up.

(Jack: 9 yrs after diagnosis with Hodgkin's lymphoma)

Louise had not initially planned to go to university, but her inability to take up a training post at the time of her diagnosis had resulted in her going to university after her recovery, thus possibly having a positive impact on her career choice:

I decided that I wasn't going to go to university, and I was sort of job hunting at the time ... I'd actually applied for a job [in] Life Assurance, which was ... I mean it's nothing like what I do now. It was just a job which would be like a traineeship I guess. And I applied for that, and I actually got told that I got accepted on the day that I was going for all my bone scans and everything. So obviously I couldn't take that ... I was absolutely adamant I was not going to university. And then ... once I finished my treatment I went down to London and did some work for the TCT, because I was ... I really wanted to get involved. And then it didn't last very long because I was extremely homesick. And my landlady ... the lady that I lived with in London – and it was only for like 4 weeks – said to me you need to ... you know if you want to get a good job you need a degree. So I just decided ... I came home and decided to do a degree. And then I went and I did my degree, and I spent 4 months living in Finland ... I think university, and certainly living abroad in Finland on my own, where I was very home-sick, completely changed [me]. I feel like I found my brain. As bad as that sounds, but I went from like a C grade student to an A grade student. And then since then I've just been like ... you know I've had the taste for it, and then I've always wanted to do well. And since then I've got my job, I work at the local council ... I've since done my postgraduate certificate in HR, and I just strive now to get the best. Even though you don't always need it, you just need a pass, but I just always want the best of the best. I'm that type of person ... So I don't ever, ever settle for second best now, ever.

(Louise: 8 yrs after diagnosis with Ewing's sarcoma)

In Chapters 5 and 6 we have already seen examples of changes in philosophy and the possibility of positive outcomes but I have left the elements of these aspects in Louise's quotation to contextualise not only how her life plans changed but how the cancer experience shaped her choices in a very positive way. We have already seen in the last chapter that Ashley and Marc had both taken on the identity of survivorship as key to their professional lives. Further to Marc's role as a motivational speaker and sponsored athlete is the follow-ing information on how his career trajectory was fundamentally changed by the illness:

Well university was delayed for a year. I was part way through an appli-cation to be a pilot in the fleet air arm, but that wasn't going to happen. I mean it impacts on me on every way. It affects my income now, in that I earn decent money doing what I do. It's telling my story, which is ... part of it is obviously getting cancer, part of it is swimming for Great Britain, or mountaineering, or whatever it is that I want to talk about. And so I guess the cancer was the turning point that set this story, as I tell it, in motion. So it affects everything ... I drive a nice car and have [a] nice house because I had cancer, that's not quite right ... I speak to the corporate world ... you name a company I've probably spoken to [it] if not that company, one that's similar or in the same industry. It's not specific to any particular industry; it's more to do ... I guess you'd call it motivational speaking.

(Marc: 21 yrs after diagnosis with osteosarcoma)

The following extract from Mary's interview brings together a number of issues that show how her life plans have been shaped and, like others who have been drawn into health-related work, she trained to be a dental nurse and also a psychotherapist. She also told me that because she had several recurrences she did not begin to think of herself as a survivor for 10 years after her initial diagnosis:

Yes, because I'd had it back I was thinking it's going to come back. So I made a lot of adjustments in my life to accommodate that: where I lived, which hospital I went to, what job I did, that I didn't have a family at that point ... I took those choices because I thought alright you know, I don't feel very well and I'm probably going to have it back – or I might have it back. I didn't stop thinking like that, and I started planning ahead and doing more long-term things when I was about 30. So that was about 9/10 years afterwards. And I actually had a bit of ... so I had a bit of a mad teenage sort of year the year I was 30. I did lots of quite whacky things. And I think it was a bit of you know ... I don't know, doing things I hadn't done. I got very into sport, because by then I started to feel well you know. I hadn't ... obviously hadn't felt very well since I was about 15, I should think, because I [was] diagnosed at 17 and I think I was in decline from about 15 onwards. And hadn't ever been very sporty at school, I was always tired. So by the time I was sort of in my late 20s–28, 29, 30– I'd taken up horse riding as a hobby, as a new thing for me. I was really into that. And I was quite fit, quite well, I looked good. I bought a sports car. I was having a nice time ... So I was sort of almost making up for lost time I think.

I had wanted to be an architect. And I had done my A levels, and I'd been to university, got a three year degree in Landscape Architecture in fact. And I wanted to be a landscape architect originally, and then an architect, but that went by the board ... I realised it was going to be a very hard slog to do what I was doing ... when I had my final do with Hodgkin's disease I'd actually got my first job in architecture. I was designing car parks of all things. And I went off sick from that, and very kindly they paid me sick pay while I was off. But I could never go back. I'd lost all my hair, I had no confidence, I felt dizzy if I stood up quickly. There was no way I could put a hard hat on and go up ladders in a very male-dominated office where I worked. I just couldn't do it. So I think I quite quickly realised I needed something I could do part time that was in a supportive environment, that I could you know pick up and put down more easily ... I mean I'd witnessed you know great things while I'd been in hospital, and I think now I want to join these people and be one of them ... I completely retrained ... and by 30, I was actually quite good at

what I was doing ... and started to think oh you know it's worth saving for a pension you know, it's worth getting a mortgage, buying a house. And started to think about a family in fact as well, which actually for me never happened. But at the time I was thinking about that sort of stuff.
(Mary: 24 years after diagnosis with Hodgkin's lymphoma)

This extract also resonates with other accounts relating to risk-taking, making up for lost time and fertility, but I have left the quote intact in order to present the material in context. Like Andrea, Mary told me that her first marriage had resulted primarily from being too hasty – another decision shaped by her illness:

We lasted 13 years – I was 34 when we divorced. But I can honestly say that going through what we went through made a massive difference ... the short answer is that we got married in the first place in haste. I think if I hadn't been ill we might have waited a year or two, and maybe we would have learnt more about each other. That's the simple answer. I think the more complex question is the fact that I became ... I changed ... I changed. I became a very needy, quite vulnerable person, and very clingy. And he of course being a pilot was in fact away quite a lot. He came out of the Air Force as a result of me being ill and did short-haul flying. And that was actually fine. It worked well. And then at 34 he joined BA. He was very good at what he did. He joined BA and became a long-haul pilot. And I couldn't cope with the separation. I just felt like my saviour had gone.
(Mary: 24 yrs after diagnosis with Hodgkin's lymphoma)

Kate had done a degree in engineering in the 1970s and subsequently found it difficult to obtain an appropriate job in engineering at graduate level. However, she felt that the deleterious effect on her 'brilliant career' was probably more to do with being a woman in a man's world at a time when women engineers were almost unheard of. Nevertheless, the illness had left her with an abiding interest in health-related issues and she had acted as a volunteer on various bodies:

I'm quite interested in health-related matters, which I wouldn't have been otherwise ... I do voluntary work for a Patient Involvement Forum ... and before that with the Community Health Council ... we visit premises and inspect them. We meet members of the public and talk about their health experiences, that kind of thing ... I [want to] put something back into the NHS ... I had a fairly rotten time when I was ill, particularly with the consultant that thought he was more important than God. God sat at his right hand. And that was in the days when consultants were like that. [You're] just a piece of meat – a patient ... and I just felt I wanted to try and, in some small way, make the experience of being ill better for people ... not so much of the medical side of it, as communication or the sort of holistic, looking after the person rather than just seeing to the illness.
(Kate: 31 yrs after diagnosis with Hodgkin's lymphoma)

Kate's motivation is similar to Bob's (see Chapter 1) in that her bad experience had motivated her to try to improve the patient experience in general. Her evocation of the consultant as a 'God-like' figure and her interpretation of patients simply being 'a piece of meat' helps us to make sense of her hatred of the word 'patient' (see last chapter). A similar motivation lay behind Phoebe's determination to work for the TCT. She had graduated from university without much idea of what she wanted to do but her experience of cancer had compelled her to try to improve that of others:

> I didn't really know what I wanted to do. I knew I kind of wanted to do something like management or something like that, but I didn't know what I wanted to do. And it just gave me a direction. And now it's made me realise that there's such a huge gap in the medical service in England for that age group and for teenagers. That's the only thing I wanted to get involved in. So I just kept writing to the Teenage Cancer Trust until they let me work for them.
>
> (Phoebe: 2 yrs after diagnosis with acinic cell carcinoma)

A much longer time after his illness than Phoebe, Richard told a very similar story which suggests that the issues remain the same and have a far-reaching and long-lasting impact on feelings about medical provision and attitudes to patients. They are directly shaped by the experience of the cancer treatment:

> You know I get angry that you know people are still misdiagnosed. I get angry that consultants still don't communicate properly ... I've always taken the view that I'm not you know a scientist or a doctor; you know I can't do anything on that side but I've always been able to raise money in the corporate sector, and that's the only contribution I can really make.
>
> (Richard: 36 yrs after diagnosis with aggressive fibro sarcoma)

Some accounts make it clear that the illness impacted in a very obvious way on a career or on educational opportunities, but Trevor could not confirm the extent to which his life plans had been shaped by the experience:

> I missed out an awful lot of fundamental stuff when I was in treatment or recovering from treatment ... potentially if that hadn't happened I probably would have done a lot better in my higher grades ... then I may have gone to university or may not, and then I may be in a different role. But at the end of the day, you know I chose a different path. I can't say that's absolutely down to you know what happened to me as a child. But there probably is some impact there, and from an educational point in terms of you know missing out a little bit of education. And it sort of maybe drives you down a different road.
>
> (Trevor: 24 yrs after diagnosis with Hodgkin's lymphoma)

The long-term financial implications

It is apparent from the earlier accounts that life plans were changed, opportunities lost – and gained – and careers shaped by the illness either directly or
indirectly. Given that the issues raised have financial implications this is the
topic to which we now turn. While it seems that Marc has succeeded financially, at least in part as a result of his cancer, this may be an unusual outcome
of the illness. For example Julie's probably more generalisable experience is
as follows:

> One thing that [got] hit quite hard and fast, was our finances ... Yes, we
> got into really serious debt through my Hodgkin's. And that had a
> knock-on effect for about 10 years ... It was the cost of illness first of all
> ... because at that time I couldn't be treated locally ... and especially
> when I had the radiotherapy ... there was a choice, I could either spend 4
> weeks going everyday back and forth ... which really wasn't an option,
> especially with Guy (son) being, you know tiny. The other option was
> that I was admitted to hospital for 4 weeks, [to] which I said 'no, I'm not
> ... no, I want to be with my child and my husband as well of course ... I
> don't want to be away from home'. So the third option was that we
> rented a flat ... and that really hit us in the pocket ... Because we had like
> ... mortgage and rent and everything. And then there was all ... there was
> a lot of travelling and everything with appointments ... John (husband)
> didn't work for a year because he was signed off because ... it hit him very
> hard all of this – harder than me ... he was signed off with stress. And yes,
> so he wasn't working for a bit. And then, oh I don't know allsorts of
> things. It just really kind of ... we just took out more and more borrow-
> ing and everything, and it just ... And then when I stopped working, it all
> kind of crashed a bit ... I mean we did have some help, like the Macmillan
> Fund helped pay for some of the flat expenses ... that did go on for a long
> time and ... added a lot to our worry and stress and everything for a long
> time afterwards and limited what we could do as well.
>
> (Julie: 15 yrs after diagnosis with Hodgkin's lymphoma)

Trevor told me that while he had been able to get a mortgage, he had been put
on higher premiums for 3 years at the outset. For Scott, who felt he needed life
insurance to cover his substantial mortgage, premiums were a great deal
higher:

> I was substantially stepping up my liability in terms of the mortgage, that
> was the first time I thought I really need to ... for my wife, to make sure
> I've got life cover. And I had to jump through a few hoops to get the
> cover, but actually I got there in the end. I do pay a premium for it in
> terms of I pay a lot more than perhaps I would had I not had any health
> issues.
>
> (Scott: 18 yrs after diagnosis with ALL)

Kelly had also been asked for a very high premium for life insurance:

> The other thing that I really struggled with, and I still don't have, is life insurance ... the quotes that I've had for life insurance, even being 6 years finished [after the illness] are just astronomical. I mean like £230 a month ... that's a third of my mortgage ... so I don't actually have life insurance, which I think is quite a dangerous thing to do but ... I can't afford to. I've got a mortgage, but that's only a recent thing ... in fact they didn't ask anything about my health. I'm sure they would have turned me down otherwise ... I think probably if I tried to apply for one now with things being much tighter, and them looking for excuses not to give them out, I'm sure they would use it.
>
> (Kelly: 7 yrs after diagnosis with non-Hodgkin's lymphoma)

Kelly was speaking to me at the time when the 'credit crunch' of 2008 was making headline news, and whether she was right or wrong about the likelihood of her being given a mortgage under that financial climate it was her belief that her illness legacy would follow her through life and continue to affect her ability to secure financial products.

John had strong feelings about the financial legacy of his illness which even 33 years later he viewed as a permanent but unseen reminder:

> Well in the early days when I first got married I couldn't get a mortgage ... and it wasn't 'til 20 years post diagnosis that I got my first mortgage. So that really had an impact. And those issues had to be addressed later in life ... I'm a little bit bitter towards the establishment for their blinkered approach to cancer patients, and the fact that you know although ... I've organised my future finances now, you know they would certainly without a shadow of a doubt be a lot healthier had I have been able to do that as a younger person ... we see this even to this very day with regards to travel insurance ... Even those patients who are potentially going to be cured, those patients who have recently finished chemotherapy and/or radiotherapy, and they'll come in and say do you have any information with regards to which companies will be more sympathetic. A lot of companies still put overloads onto their premiums for cancer patients; because it's so easy, and ... I personally see it as extortion. But it's so easy to say to a cancer patient well you know you're more of a risk so we're going to charge you more money ... it's that permanent and unseen reminder.
>
> (John: 33 yrs after diagnosis with Hodgkin's lymphoma)

Richard's account is similar to John's in many ways and emphasises the lasting and long-term financial impact. It also makes clear the point that even without the continuing pain as a reminder of his cancer, Richard's working life was to some extent shaped and governed by his constant awareness that he had to compensate for the financial insecurity resulting from the cancer:

I mean we couldn't get a mortgage to start with because … it hadn't been in remission for 5 years. So that side of it was difficult. You know life insurance, those sorts of things, travel insurance. But you know you just battle on and find a way of doing certain things. And eventually you know we got there and … but certainly I think I got very, very focused on, you know maximising my career so that we could have that financial stability, not knowing what the long-term prognosis really was, or you know the damage that had been done.

(Richard: 36 yrs after diagnosis with aggressive fibro sarcoma)

Richard's illness also changed his life plans in that it precipitated his decision and his wife's to have children earlier than they might otherwise have done. His choice of the words 'stupidly' and 'irresponsible' are interesting in that clearly many years after the event and seen in the light of a more 'mature' attitude they might, as a couple, have made a different decision. Yet the age and life stage once again have had the effect of changing the course of lives at that crucial moment when such decisions are made:

We actually started a family quite young because you know very stupidly we looked at the future and thought it was quite uncertain to me, so why don't we start a family now. You know a young wife potentially [would] have to bring up two young kids on her own, without me around, and without any life insurance. Which when you look back was pretty irresponsible. But that's how we thought at the time. And so you know our children are quite grown up now.

(Richard: 36 yrs after diagnosis with aggressive fibro sarcoma)

One possibly unexpected financial legacy is that a person diagnosed with cancer in early adulthood may not expect to have to provide for his/her old age and may as a consequence be left without the resources to do so:

I mean I never … I never took out a [pension] … I don't get a pension with my job. And I never took out a personal pension plan. I never thought I'd get to 60, 65. I mean come on – nobody was telling me I'd ever get to that age and I presumed I wouldn't. I've got to 54, and I've suddenly taken out a pension plan, because I thought hang on I'm going to make it to 60, I'm going to make it to 65. I've made my retirement age at 65. You know I'm going to make it to that and it's only in a way since I turned 50 that it's even occurred to me; I'm going to get old. I'm not going to die young. I'm not young now.

(Gillian: 34 yrs after diagnosis with Hodgkin's lymphoma)

Summary

Without doubt all the participants quoted thus far have had the course of their lives changed in far-reaching ways as a result of the illness. However long since the illness all participants – those quoted and those who have not been – indicated both implicitly and explicitly that the life stage at which they had been diagnosed had altered their life course, their options and their choices. In other words, at this juncture the diagnosis of cancer has a far-reaching and lasting impact on the remainder of life.

However, there appear to be a number of critical factors that contribute to the legacy being interpreted and experienced as positive or negative. There are accounts of positive and beneficial outcomes, careers that have been kick-started by a response to the cancer experience or chance meetings that have resulted indirectly from the illness. It is also important to remember how many people in the last chapter said that their lives had been positively affected. Nevertheless, the accounts are also permeated with stories of loss and disappointment – as we can see in this chapter – there are also those who feel that their life chances have been constrained and damaged as a result of the illness. So what are the contributory factors that shape the future?

Participants such as Majad, Maz and Meg felt that their lives – both personal and working – had been blighted by the illness. They had all been unable to pursue their chosen careers or remain in employment and this had had implications for their quality of life on a variety of fronts – financial, emotional and social. These participants had been manual workers and thus it is unsurprising that their strength and stamina having been affected by the illness, they had needed to find alternative employment or remain unemployed. However, there are also examples of other participants who had planned, for example, sporting careers and who also found they had to reinvent their life plans and yet did so with more success and a more positive attitude. Was this because of the social and cultural capital available to them? If that is the case then it is vital at the time of the diagnosis and treatment that the social context of patients' lives is taken into account. Does this phenomenon take us back to the concept of the 'inverse care law' first invoked by Tudor Hart in 1971?

> The inverse care law was suggested thirty years ago by Julian Tudor Hart in a paper for *The Lancet*, to describe a perverse relationship between the need for health care and its actual utilisation. In other words, those who most need medical care are least likely to receive it. Conversely, those with least need of health care tend to use health services more (and more effectively).
>
> (Appleby and Deeming 2001: 37)

If it is indeed the case that some survivors of adolescent and young adult cancer are doubly disadvantaged by life chances because of their circumstances, it seems even more imperative that the setting of care should be in an age-appropriate environment where such effects can be mitigated. My previous research (Grinyer 2007) suggests strongly that this is where a multidisciplinary team, expert not only in the medical care but also in social, educational and financial issues, is best equipped to maximise the chances of a beneficial outcome in its wider sense.

However, while such an approach in an age-specific care setting may alleviate some of the longer-term educational and employment challenges, it is likely to do little to impact on the services provided by the financial sector commented on earlier. Indeed Soliman and Agresta (2008) suggest that financial assistance for survivors in this age group needs to be an integral part of a survivorship plan that requires a co-ordinated effort from social workers. As Hoffmann (2007) says an evaluation of employment and insurance needs should begin at diagnosis and team-based long-term support in managing these issues should be available. Difficulty in obtaining life insurance, travel insurance, mortgages and other such financial products needs to be addressed on behalf of this increasing number of people who it appears can be disadvantaged throughout their lives. Perhaps if they are recognised as a cohort whose illness has distinct life stage effects it will enhance the chances of mitigating long-term disadvantage.

Key points

Life plans

* Life plans are seriously disrupted
* Education is interrupted
* Careers can be terminated – particularly those that involve a need for stamina or athleticism
* Confidence may be adversely impacted
* Unwise choices might be made as result

However:

* Such disruptions can result in new opportunities
* Contingent encounters may shape life in a positive way
* Careers can be enhanced or result from the illness

Finance

* Long-term financial hardship can result from the illness
* Time away from work is costly
* Travel and accommodation for treatment at a distant centre can be costly
* Mortgages can be more expensive
* Life insurance can be hard to find and expensive
* Old age may not be anticipated and catered for
* Careers started late may never provide the financial security from which early starters benefit

8 The impact on fertility

It has become apparent throughout the preceding chapters that long-term survivorship from cancer in adolescence and young adulthood has far-reaching and lasting consequences: physical, emotional, psychological and on planning for the future. All these aspects are brought together in a single issue that can be experienced as a result of either the illness or its treatment – that is the risk of infertility.

As Levitt and Eshelman (2008) argue, pubertal development and the assurance of future fertility are important milestones in adolescence and young adulthood yet cancer treatments can result in infertility for both young men and young women. As this age group are unlikely to have already become parents, or to have completed their families (Grinyer 2007) the prospect of infertility can be a cause of additional distress and anxiety.

The threats to infertility are well documented; according to Reebals *et al.* (2006) between 15–30 per cent of cancer survivors are left permanently sterile following therapy. In addition, Wallace and Brougham (2005) say that gonadal damage and resulting infertility can be caused, not only by chemotherapy and radiotherapy, but also by the disease itself. An early menopause may also be experienced by women (Schover 2007). Schover cites the trend for delaying families until women are in their 30s as a salient factor in cancer survivorship for women who have yet to bear children. However, while there may be a recent and increasing trend for women who choose to delay starting a family, Schover does not mention the impact on much younger women who would have been even less likely to have completed or even started their families in their teenage years even without the more recent trend for giving birth to first children at a later age.

How well the young people are prepared for the loss of fertility, in terms of both information and the offer of fertility preservation, at the time of diagnosis, varies according to the expertise and willingness of health professionals to engage with them in a discussion about their options (Shaw *et al.* 2004, Reebals *et al.* 2006).

The option for young men to bank sperm is comparatively straightforward yet as Schover (2007) says the most common reason given for the failure to bank sperm is a lack of timely information with only half of the sample of young men in a survey recalling the option being offered to them. For females the preservation of fertility is more complex (Levitt and Eshelman 2008). One option is the collection of mature oocytes that can be used for In Vitro Fertilisation (IVF) and subsequent embryo cryopreservation. However, the option of ovarian tissue harvesting is not suitable for all patients (Wallace and Brougham 2005); the urgency of treatment may preclude the invasive and time-consuming nature of the intervention. Yet, despite the threat to fertility for both males and females, Zebrack (2006) reports that the prospect of infertility may come as a surprise to young adult cancer survivors who do not recall being told that their treatment might affect their future fertility.

This chapter looks at the impact of fertility issues on the lives of long-term survivors. Several outcomes are represented in the following accounts from 1) those who have had concerns that their fertility has been affected, 2) those whose fertility has been affected, and 3) those whose assumptions of infertility have been proved wrong. However, whatever the eventual outcome, it is clear from the ways in which fertility issues are addressed that this is a significant issue of considerable concern for both male and female survivors.

Concerns about fertility and the genetic legacy

We begin with Vicky who said that fertility was a deep and ongoing concern for her. Vicky did not know her fertility status but was concerned that she might have become infertile as a result of her treatment for ovarian cancer or because of the illness itself. However, she acknowledged that it was only 4 years after her diagnosis that she was feeling strong enough to address the issue and her fears. The extract I have selected from her interview is lengthy because of the compelling way in which it conveys the depth of her concern, the difficulty she has had in accessing information and advice and the lack of understanding that can be shown by medical professionals:

> After the operation and everything had happened, I wasn't feeling emotionally stable enough to deal with the fact that I might be infertile. So I was put on the pill and then it was only last August that I decided that I wanted to come off the pill and see if I could have natural periods – which I have been having ... until about 2 months ago when for some reason it stopped ... As soon as it happened [fertility] was the biggest concern and in the last few years that's been the major concern, but I feel that I haven't really had anyone that I could talk to about it ... the consultant has been fantastic ... I have three monthly meetings with him, where he checks my blood and he does scans ... but it's never actually been possible to talk to him about fertility options, what I could do? He hasn't really known who to pass me on to. I just don't think that it's within his knowledge ... I would've liked to have been able to see a specialist in the area ... because obviously like time's ticking ... I had six periods ... I thought this could be my chance, I might be fertile. But ... he wanted to see whether they

were regular I just felt that in the 6 months where I was having regular periods, something maybe could have been done then. Because obviously I have no idea who I need to see or what exactly is happening.

I went to see my GP and I think I'd just been on antibiotics or something, and he said to me, 'Oh do you realise that this could affect you know, the pill that you're on. So it might not work.' And I said, 'Yes I realise that.' Then he looked at my notes better and said, 'Oh yes, but that's not going to affect you anyway is it with your history.' And I just feel that ... he was extremely insensitive ... I said look this is a really sensitive situation and ... I would like to talk to someone about that. He didn't refer me to ... anyone either ... I just wish that there was some way in which I could talk to someone about exactly what the things were that I could do now.

I would have welcomed some fertility advice or some advice from a female doctor straight afterwards ... because then she would have said 3 years ago to me, 'Look stop being silly, you know come off the pill and see whether you have proper periods ...' you know 3 years ago rather than waiting until now. But because I was kind of left to my own devices as far as that goes. Because as long as my specialist saw that my blood was okay and everything ... every 3 months, he didn't actually say to me maybe you should be thinking about what ... the remnant of your ovary's doing. But I guess that's because that's just not his side of it. But it would have been good to have seen a female doctor or nurse or a specialist ... and someone like you could go and talk to [someone who] wasn't like my GP who would forget who I was and start talking about something else, and then realise what kind of treatment I'd been through or whatever. Because I thought every time I went to see him, and I thought oh I'll ask him about coming off the pill and everything, he was just not at all ... or he just wasn't very nice about it. He wasn't very compassionate at all.

I guess it's made me a bit bitter ... [and] angry about people who maybe are extremely fertile and don't think about it ... I guess it affected me a lot, of the effect that it had on my mum ... she feels that there's nothing she can do anymore because now she's had the hysterectomy. I think when it first happened there was talk of her freezing some of her eggs ... I feel that everything could have been looked into in much more detail there and then. Because nobody ever spoke to me about freezing eggs, about whether I was producing eggs at the time or anything like that.

(Vicky: 5 yrs after diagnosis with ovarian cancer)

While Vicky's medical care was, according to her, excellent and her cancer had been treated successfully, none of those involved in her care had either much interest in, or any expert knowledge of, fertility issues. She felt let down by a system that had left her unprepared and ill informed and there is a strong sense of her fear that time is slipping away and a possible window of opportunity is being lost. Her resulting distress and the detrimental impact on her emotional well-being are understandable. The frustration at her lack of progress through a system that has not prioritised her possibly limited potential to conceive is clear, yet she does not know where to turn. The support services and follow-up care are concerned with preventing recurrence not maximising the chances of conception. This is clearly a life stage related issue that would be inapplicable to a childhood survivor at the same stage of recovery, and possibly of much less relevance to an older woman who had completed her family. In contrast, Kelly had apparently been given more information and had undergone a number of fertility tests yet she too was uncertain about her fertility status:

> Well, the tumour that I had was quite big when they found it, so they basically said we need to start treatment straight away. Are you in a relationship? I said no, so they carried straight on. So I wasn't offered any fertility treatment at all, basically because they said they needed to get started … so when I finished obviously I asked will I be okay. And then said well as far as we can tell you're okay but you need to have tests … I waited about 4 years until I did anything about it – I think out of fear. And I've had all the tests that I can have, apart from actually trying to get pregnant. And they've all come back fine. But what I have been told is that I should probably try and have children around or before 30 … because I might experience an early menopause, but obviously people are having children later … I might not have wanted to have children until sort of mid 30s. And that's less of an option now … if I want them I need to try earlier.
>
> (Kelly: 7 yrs after diagnosis with non-Hodgkin's lymphoma)

Kelly's account again raises the issue of life stage, as she says many young women are now opting to become mothers later in life after establishing a career; and of course others in this age group may not be in a relationship or in the kind of relationship where children are an option. Kelly also said that the prospect of infertility and an early menopause had precipitated – early in her relationship when they should just have been having fun – the kind of conversation that would normally take place much later. At the time of the interview Vicky and Kelly were unaware whether or not their fertility had been damaged, but Andrea knew that she had been made infertile by her treatment and told me the following story:

> Because of all the chemotherapy and then the body radiation treatment I had, and it was whole body radiation, so it affected my endocrine system, it affected my hormones … about 2 years after I'd finished all my treatment for the leukaemia that they realised that my hormones were imbalanced, and they did tests, one thing and another, and they found that my thyroid was underactive. And of course they knew that the treatment had wiped out my ovaries … I'm on like HRT, because it's as if my body's gone through the change you see.
>
> (Andrea: 21 yrs after diagnosis with acute myeloid leukaemia)

I was aware at the interview that Andrea had a young son and asked her if the treatment and its after effects had made conception problematic:

> I knew I couldn't [have a baby] from having my bone marrow transplant I knew that that would be it. That the radiation treatment would basically damage my ovaries, and there wouldn't be any chance of it. But at the time of going through that, I mean of course at 18 that wasn't really something in my mind … I don't remember being sat down and told exactly. But I somehow knew, and I somehow feel that it obviously came via my mum … with her being an ex-nurse she knew a lot about it … for a long time after it was … it wasn't a big issue, but then of course when I met my first husband, and we got married, we obviously talked about it, and thought about it, and it wasn't a great big issue to us, but we knew that there was an option of having treatment with an egg donor you see. Whether … and at that time they weren't even sure whether that would work, because they didn't know … there was no reason why I couldn't carry a child, but there was no way of them really knowing whether it would work. So then with my first husband we did put our names down on the egg donor list, but shortly after that things started getting you know, bad … and we went our separate ways. After my first marriage … I met Andy … it didn't bother him at all … that I couldn't have children. It wasn't an issue. But as we sort of grew together we decided that … we knew that we could try this treatment, having an egg donor. And we decided that if we didn't try it we'd regret it … we had an anonymous donor matched up. And of course it's the sort of treatment that you know, you're very lucky if it all works first time, and you could be going through it a few times. We were lucky enough to have it all funded. [It would it have cost] over £3,000 [for] each attempt … they only actually had one embryo they could use … So they implanted it, and it was just pot luck basically.
>
> (Andrea: 21 yrs after diagnosis with acute myeloid leukaemia)

That embryo turned out to be Andrea's son Callum, 5 years old at the time of the interview:

> He was determined from the start. One embryo, first time, we were really lucky … He's 5 now. So you know we obviously feel very, very lucky to have him … and he's absolutely treasured. He's gorgeous. Yes, bless him. So you know it's … he feels … because I mean I carried him for 9 months you know.
>
> (Andrea: 21 yrs after diagnosis with acute myeloid leukaemia)

But Andrea went on to tell me that the pregnancy had not been entirely without problems and that the diabetes she developed was related to her earlier treatment for the cancer:

It was a fairly hard pregnancy because I got diabetes very early on ... because of all that (the treatment) ... [it] was fairly bad diabetes as far as it goes. I had to inject insulin and everything. And they didn't think that it would go afterwards, but now fortunately it has gone.

(Andrea: 21 yrs after diagnosis with acute myeloid leukaemia)

As with Vicky and Andrea, for Katie fertility had not been her primary concern for at the time of diagnosis:

At the time when I got the cancer I wasn't bothered because I was only 19, I wasn't feeling particularly maternal. I had asked the question, just so that I knew because they had removed one of the ovaries, but you know they said well as far as we're concerned there's no problem. It was probably in my early 20s when I started thinking actually yes I would like kids. And when I met my husband, he definitely wanted kids so we had to sort of discuss it ... I'd had enough of hospitals, and also because of the emotional trauma of IVF we said we won't go through IVF, we will try for our own, but if we can't have our own we'll just adopt ... but in the end, I actually got pregnant within about 2 or 3 months of trying.

(Katie: 13 yrs after diagnosis with ovarian cancer)

For Rowena, the knowledge that she would be unable to bear a child was mitigated to some extent by the fact that the man she was to marry had children already, thus she was philosophical about the relationship she had been able to establish as a step-parent:

Fortunately I'd already met my husband – well he wasn't my husband then – and he already had his three children. So I think that lessened the blow slightly. I mean obviously it's always a blow when you get told definitively sorry you're never going to be ... you know be able to have children. But it didn't impact a great deal on me, because I already had three stepchildren. And in hindsight you know maybe that was the way it should be, because that way I love my stepchildren. They're with us, you know a lot of the time they don't live with us permanently ... I mean they're a lot older now but ... had we had a child between us, you know you just never know how you would have felt about that child that was your own against your stepchildren. So in hindsight I've always said to my husband it's fate that I met you – that you already had children. And yes we would probably have had children together, but it wasn't a huge blow. It didn't, you know make me really upset. It was just that you've taken that choice away and I don't like that, but I accept that if I've got to go through this treatment then that's one of the side effects.

(Rowena: 12 yrs after first diagnosis with Hodgkin's lymphoma)

Rowena comments on how much she dislikes the fact that her choice has been taken away, but her stepchildren have clearly mitigated the loss she would have otherwise felt. It seems significant that Katie and her husband had decided that if a pregnancy did not result without medical intervention they would adopt. Katie in her own words 'had enough of hospitals' and was unwilling to subject herself to yet more tests and invasive procedures so evocative of her illness and which would carry a significant emotional cost. At the time I interviewed her, Katie had given birth to a second baby which, as with the first, resulted from a pregnancy that had not required any medical assistance. However, her second baby had health problems:

> The second [baby], our son's been recently diagnosed with muscular dystrophy. Which we don't think is connected but there's always a possibility it's connected with having had the chemo ... they're trying to suss it out because it's only recent, there's no family history. They can't isolate the exact bit of genetics that's caused it with him at the moment. So they're sort of going through that process, which is going to take a while ... we talked to the genetics people, they don't think it's connected, but obviously they can't rule it out ... I think ... if there'd been hints that 'oh if you have a child it might be disabled' ... then I'd probably feel guilty that 'oh well I went ahead and tried anyway'. But I didn't, we didn't have any idea that any of this could happen ... if they did ... say it was to do with the chemo ... I might feel a bit more annoyed about having had the cancer, if that makes sense ... [and] wish it hadn't have happened a bit more.
>
> (Katie: 13 yrs after diagnosis with ovarian cancer)

Her son's medical condition could not be attributed to Katie's illness with any certainty. However, it is clear that if this were the case, or had Katie been warned of complications and proceeded in any case, her guilt would be considerable and the emotional legacy of the illness would be greater. At the time of my interview with Janet, her daughter was a young adult herself. Janet told me that a problem with her daughter's lymph glands in her groin had resulted in one of her legs being affected by a distressing lymphoedema. Although Janet had been assured that there was no hereditary connection to her own lymphoma, she could not help but connect the two lymphatic conditions and felt that the problem her daughter had been born with might have some connection to her lymphoma:

> Funnily enough my daughter was actually born with a condition which is ... it's a problem with her lymph glands as well, although they do assure me it's completely coincidental.
>
> (Janet: 27 yrs after diagnosis with Hodgkin's lymphoma)

Like Katie, Janet spoke of the guilt she would feel if her own illness had caused her daughter's condition. Thus it seems that for those women who do give birth there may be a tendency to attribute any illnesses in their children to their own cancers, even if they are assured by the health professionals that this is not the case. While Lesley was not worried about her daughter's health she did have a concern over her fertility:

> I do sometimes have a little thought that I wonder if Jade will be able to conceive naturally. I don't know where that comes from. That's my only thought.
>
> (Lesley: 18 yrs after diagnosis with Hodgkin's lymphoma)

Interestingly Lesley, who also had a son, was not concerned about his fertility though she acknowledged that her position was not informed by any medical evidence, the illness had left her with what might be deemed an irrational fear. After all she was the one whose fertility had been compromised by her treatment yet she had conceived naturally on two occasions. Yet while her daughter had not been exposed to any radiotherapy, she still feared for her fertility, but her son, whom it could be interpreted would be at similar risk should there be any, she had no concerns over. We can see that even 18 years after the illness its legacy still haunted what was, in other respects, a happy family situation.

Debbie had given birth to two children though she had not become pregnant easily and remained uncertain if that was because of the cancer or her treatment for it. Nevertheless, the legacy of her lymphoma resulted in post-natal complications:

> After my son ... my first baby was delivered, it was a very, very difficult delivery – very traumatic. And it was all a bit of a sort of cock-up really, because the midwife looking after me hadn't read my notes properly. The consultant had said if I showed any signs of an infection he wanted me treated immediately and aggressively ... [because of] the lymphoma – just in case and ... they hadn't read that. So anyway, to cut a long story short, I ended up with a massive pelvic haematoma that then got infected ... So I was very, very poorly afterwards. And it took about six to eight weeks to actually heal up properly [I needed] bucket loads of antibiotics ... I was 30, so I was sort of 5 years post-treatment. And they'd said to me they didn't want me to have a baby before then and that any infection should be treated aggressively at that time, because I probably was a still a bit immuno-suppressed ... unfortunately, because they were very busy, nobody really picked up on that ... 'til after I'd already got infected and was catheterised and you know, I mean it was just ... it was a mess.
>
> (Debbie: 22 yrs after diagnosis with Hodgkin's lymphoma)

Here it seems that Debbie's illness history was not taken into account during the immediate post-natal period, suggesting no continuing care pathway or effective communication was in place between medical specialisms.

Unexpected fertility

While the accounts up to this point have related to women who had either feared infertility, been uncertain of their fertility status or who had experienced difficulties with pregnancy or its aftermath, Elaine B's unexpected discovery that she had retained her fertility had far-reaching consequences:

> They actually did tests ... and they said I could never conceive, and never carry children ... they did blood tests and tested my hormones, and did all sorts of things. And then tested my pituitary gland, and my ovaries, and things like that. And they said that there was nothing ... my body wasn't sending signals at all, in any way ... I didn't find out [I was pregnant] until I was five and a half months pregnant. [I was] absolutely thrilled. Absolutely. For starters ... well I went to the doctor's thinking I had a lump in my stomach ... and because I was told I could never have children; I never had a period or things like that. And I was on HRT tablets, because I'd started a menopause thing, because ... nothing was working. So I was on HRT tablets for a number of years ... and then five and a half months pregnant I went to my normal GP, and I said there's a lump in my stomach. So ... he felt, and then he went out the room, and he came in with his stethoscope, and he said, 'Do you know what that is?' And he said, 'It's a foetal heartbeat,' he said, 'you're at least 20 weeks gone' and I was 24 weeks pregnant. They [the oncologists] were surprised. They didn't know how I'd conceived, or what had happened.
> (Elaine B: 15 yrs after diagnosis with Hodgkin's lymphoma)

It is clear that Elaine B had been delighted by her pregnancy and loved being a mother, yet having assumed that she was infertile she had told her partner, the baby's father, that she could not have children. He had not reacted well to the unexpected pregnancy; as she told me: 'Well it was [a] long-term [relationship] until the pregnancy ... we were dating just over a year. But when I told him he scarpered, so I've never seen him since.' While in Elaine B's case it was her unanticipated pregnancy that heralded her boyfriend's departure, the prospect of infertility can have the same effect. I use Gillian's account as a case study example of the unexpected consequences and outcomes that can have long-term consequences:

> I did have to sign to say that the treatment would more than likely leave me sterile. And then when it reoccurred in '75 I had chemotherapy. My boyfriend at the time, he ran, I never saw him again. I didn't see him for the dust. He just went. And then my parents had a friend who came to see this you know, very sick daughter. And he's 7 years older than me. But on my 21st birthday we were getting engaged ... But the day before my 21st birthday was when I found the second lump ... So I had to tell him on my 21st birthday, look before you give me the ring I've got to tell you it's all

come back again … It wasn't a possibility it was a fact. 'You will not have children' and that's actually really how it was put to me. It would make me sterile the treatment. And in fact when I got married I was going to have it taken out of the … you know the old fashioned service, but you know about 'issue', I wanted that taken out. And I simply said I can't have children. And the minister actually said well look you know, we'll do everything we can so that you can adopt. So he said leave it in, you know he said I can't take it out, but just think that you might be able to adopt. So it was very much … I know most women can't tell whether they can have children, but I mean the fact that there was a high possibility I wouldn't, he [my husband] was very understanding.

So I got married in '76, in 1979 I went to them and I said can I … look I know its highly unlikely I'll have a baby, but can I try? Is there any reason why I can't try? And they said 'no, come back come back to us in 3 years and ask the same question'. And I was very studiously using family planning and everything else. And despite all that, despite the fact I'd had radiotherapy, chemotherapy, was using family planning, I actually got pregnant … within a few weeks of being told not to … they did offer me a termination. It wasn't an option as far as I was concerned. But that was more for my own health apparently than for the foetus. I went on and had a very healthy little boy, and then a few years after that we decided 'come on look, we were lucky that time, we better start trying for a second one'.

(Gillian: 34 yrs after diagnosis with Hodgkin's lymphoma)

Gillian's unexpected fertility brought great joy to a marriage that had been undertaken with the expectation that adoption would be the only way to have children. While the women cited thus far had been told that they could face the prospect of infertility, Janet had not been warned at the time of her treatment that she might be infertile as a result. It was only when she was trying to become pregnant that she was told that this would be 'impossible'. However, she subsequently went on to confound the medical predictions by conceiving two children naturally:

So it was only … after I got married and started to try for a family that they actually said well you won't have children … when I was, you know trying and went to see a gynaecologist, and then they said well you won't have children, you've had chemotherapy … so it was really quite marvellous that I had actually had my daughter, Laura … And then I went for a check-up … one of my annual check-ups, and the doctor said have you got any children. I said yes I've got a 2 year old … And he 'Impossible, impossible, you couldn't have had a child'. Yes, but I have. And then when I back for my next appointment a year later, I'd actually had my second daughter. And I thought I hope it's the same man, because I'll tell him I'm having another one actually.

(Janet: 27 yrs after diagnosis with Hodgkin's lymphoma)

Lisa told me a very similar story about her two children having been conceived without medical assistance after she had been told she would be infertile:

> I was told definitely I wouldn't be able to have children ... because I had high-dose chemotherapy as part of my treatment ... we were in a trial – one of these trials with the chemotherapy ... obviously they talk about the implications ... and one of the implications would be there's very much the likelihood of me not being able to have children. So that was a bit of a shock, because my husband and I hadn't even married a year by the time this had all happened, being diagnosed. But at the time, you know my life was more important than children ... Obviously my views completely changed on that afterwards ... that [was] more upsetting for me than having the disease. We were looking at fertility treatment. I was looking to have egg donation, and I'd signed up with quite a few of the centres. So I had a strategy of how I was going to cope with it. That seemed to help me. And then bizarrely when I was due to go on a ... it was like a trial run of the drug to see how my womb got to the right thickness to have a fertilised egg basically put back in, to make sure it was the right thickness. Like when you're having a normal period. I wasn't having any periods then. And they put me on a regime of drugs to stimulate this, and then bizarrely it was like the next month we conceived naturally ... which shocked a number of people. My local hospital, from a fertility angle, my consultant haematologist, and the couple of hospitals I was under, they were absolutely delighted.
>
> (Lisa: 9 yrs after diagnosis with non-Hodgkin's lymphoma)

One very revealing comment made by Lisa is that at the time of her diagnosis and treatment the preservation of her life was of paramount importance – over and above the chance of having children – but that 'obviously' later this view changed completely. Lisa was already married when diagnosed, yet even at this stage in life the importance of her fertility being compromised was not the main concern. If this is the case for a newly married woman, the chances are that the significance of infertility may not be appreciated fully by women at the younger end of the age range. However (in contrast) for Louise it had been a concern, and she had had eggs harvested before treatment as she was warned she would become infertile, but she too had conceived naturally and had therefore not needed to use her stored eggs:

> I was told that because I'd be having so much chemo, and it would be such a high dosage of it, that there was a very good possibility that my eggs ... that I might not be able to have children.
>
> (Louise: 8 yrs after treatment with Ewing's sarcoma)

Unlike some of the other women who have said that it was only some time after their diagnosis and into their recovery that they began to be anxious about fertility, for Lesley it had been an overriding concern from the outset:

> They told me it would [affect my fertility] That was the most upsetting thing for me. That was worse than being told I had cancer for me … They told me there would be a 40 per cent chance I wouldn't have children. My partner at the time – who's my husband now – sort of took it positively and said well at least there's a 60 per cent chance that you can. But I found that really hard to deal with, because I'd always wanted children. But as it turned out I finished my treatment in the December, didn't have any periods at all, and fell pregnant with my daughter in the April … completely unexpectedly. I didn't even know I was pregnant 'til I was about 4 months pregnant, because I'd got no sort of symptoms that I recognised. So that was obviously an absolute blessing. And then I think I had one or two periods after my daughter, and 17 months later gave birth to my son … [My menopause] kind of started then and there. I didn't really have periods again after the children, and one or two in between the children.
>
> (Lesley: 18 yrs after diagnosis with Hodgkin's lymphoma)

Nevertheless, despite the positive outcome for Lesley having had two children naturally, she was upset at the way in which the issue had been dealt with at the time and the lack of preparation or support she had been offered:

> I don't think he was going to tell me … but I asked the question, because obviously I must have read somewhere at the time that cancer treatment could cause infertility … and he gave me the sort of 60/40 split. But that was it, I was given no sort of … what options there might be, which I think would probably have helped me a little bit at that time. You know there was no chance of freezing embryos or anything like that, no chance of freezing eggs. There was absolutely nothing. He didn't go into any options at all. So I didn't … I felt that there was not even a little flicker of hope for me at that time, which was quite hard.
>
> (Lesley: 18 yrs after diagnosis with Hodgkin's lymphoma)

Mary's account of the choices and opportunities she had been given to increase her chances of motherhood indicate insensitivity to the emotional effects of the illness. We remember from Chapter 3 that Mary had recently been diagnosed with breast cancer resulting from the radiotherapy she received for her cancer:

> With my first husband, in fact yes a sorry tale really. The chemotherapy I had in 1988 … I was told it would make me sterile. But it didn't, so I got pregnant quite … just immediately afterwards, which was unplanned … it was a bit of a miracle really. But then we lost that baby. We had a

miscarriage early on, which was extremely painful and upsetting. And after that we vowed you know for sort of a long time that we would not put ourselves through that. And in fact by the time we'd started thinking of doing something about it in our early 30s, in fact that was when our marriage ended ... I've been to see various gynaecologists along the way and said 'oh I think I'd like to do frozen embryos because I don't want to miss the boat'. And they just didn't get it. They kept saying to me in my late 20s 'oh you know have a baby now'. We don't do frozen embryos for people who haven't got cancer. And I was saying but you don't under-stand, it's too early for me, I'm just enjoying myself. So that was never offered and we never did it. And then our marriage ended.

Then I married again with the intention of sort of trying for a family. And we did a bit. And I suppose you know late 30s, and we're busy, and it hasn't happened. And in fact now at sort of 41 I'm just obviously just now going through the whole experience all over again. In October I was offered an emergency cycle of IVF. And in fact haven't taken it up, because we got to the final moment and they said oh you know, sorry but because you're 41 you've got to pay £3,000. If you were 39 you could have it for nothing ... So I actually turned round and told them to fuck off. And by this stage at 41 it's actually too late and now I'm facing what I'm facing now with the breast cancer, it is too late. So the boat has been missed. That's not to say I haven't had plenty of choices along the way. I could have gone for it and tried a bit harder. But somehow it just didn't seem the most important thing. And it hasn't happened ... some days I'm fine about it, on occasions I can get very low about it ... certainly regret, yes, regret I suppose at not getting on with it. But somehow the time never felt right, and that was because I was busy catching up on all the years I felt I'd missed out on.

(Mary: 24 yrs after diagnosis with Hodgkin's lymphoma)

It seems particularly relevant that Mary's decision to delay a pregnancy was related to what she acknowledged in the last chapter as 'making up for lost time' at a crucial stage in her late teens and early 20s. However, Mary's reluctance to become a patient again and to feel sick also contributed, more than 20 years after her diagnosis, to her ambivalence over pregnancy:

It was actually for me definitely one of the reasons ... why I didn't ever get round to having a baby, [I] could not bear the thought of being sick. Morning sickness ... [I couldn't] bear having pain and sickness again. And that was even 20 years on ... I hate going to the doctor ... I hate going to the doctor, I hate being a patient, making a fuss. I hardly ever go; And that's partly also why I didn't pursue the fertility treatment, because the few times I did go to see a gynaecologist to get some advice, I so hated being a patient that I just walked out. I just ... oh I'm not doing this; I'm certainly not having IVF you know. And yet now I look back and think well goodness me IVF is nothing compared to what I'm going through now [treatment for breast cancer]. But I just couldn't bear it.

(Mary: 24 yrs after diagnosis with Hodgkin's lymphoma)

Mary and her husband had been accepted as foster parents but since she had been recently diagnosed with grade 3 breast cancer they had been taken off the approved list of foster parents (see Chapter 3). At the time of the interview she was about to begin 8 months of chemotherapy and would have to be 2 years clear before once again being accepted as a foster parent.

The male experience

So far in this chapter we have heard only from women participants, but the men too were affected by the threat of infertility. Greg was the father of three young children at the time of the interview, thus his fertility was not in question, yet he could reflect on the anxieties the prospect of infertility had caused him:

I think I was hugely worried about it to be honest. I've always really liked kids. I've always really wanted kids … they'd said to me at 12 that you probably wouldn't be able to have [children] … And then it wasn't just one batch, it was sort of 3 or 4 batches of the thing [chemotherapy] they said was probably going to stop it … I had a bit of a descent for about 8 years in terms of what I did. Drinking, smoking, drug taking, etcetera, that sort of thing. And I think you can, although it would probably have stopped anyway, based on the fact that having a child is something that makes you not want to do that. The discovery that I could actually have a child, I think was probably just as big an impact on why that sort of attitude changed because suddenly the thing that you thought that you couldn't have that was going to be the one thing that you really wanted to have. Suddenly there was there an option again and so really the sort of lack concern and interest about your own well-being suddenly went out the window. I generally want to be healthy and fit and just become strong so that I'm, you know that, a good person to be as it were.

(Greg: 19 yrs after diagnosis with osteosarcoma)

In the chapter on risk-taking we saw that Greg identified himself as a risk taker and it is interesting to note here that it seems to be parenthood that made him revaluate the way he was living his life. He had not felt a duty to value his life simply because it had been saved; indeed it seems that the risks he took with his health in relationship to smoking suggest a certain recklessness that only being a parent mitigated.

Huxley had been warned that he would probably be infertile, yet he had parented two children naturally and greatly valued his good fortune:

And I feel very blessed with what's happened to me in my life because originally they said you've not got a lot of chance of having kids because of ... what's happened to you. And then I've got two beautiful children [who] are 12 and 8, so that's really nice.

(Huxley: 18 after diagnosis with acute lymphoblastic leukaemia)

Trevor's account was very similar to Huxley's; he had been warned that his fertility might be impaired. However, he had not been given the opportunity to bank sperm at the time. As a result, Trevor and his wife had opted for IVF treatment that had cost a great deal of money, but events subsequently took an unexpected turn:

For our first child we had IVF, because basically I had an extremely low sperm count, and the only ... pretty much the only thing that you could put that down to was my treatment. That time of my life, you know when I was basically developing ... I can't remember what they called it. When your testicles were basically either they were ... they didn't develop properly or killed off or whatever. [IVF] was actually very successful first time, yes. And you know from an IVF point of view, if it's a boy problem it's relatively easy. And then since then we've actually gone on to conceive naturally ... which is quite a surprise, but ... we've got another one due in July.

(Trevor: 24 yrs after diagnosis with Hodgkin's lymphoma)

Like the women who were concerned that their children's health had been affected by their illness or treatment, Ben was anxious that the fact that his wife had recently had a miscarriage was in some way related to his cancer. I spoke to Ben before his outpatient's clinic appointment and he told me that this was something that he was going to ask the consultant about:

Well I've been thinking about starting a family, and my wife actually got pregnant not long after we got married so I thought oh yes everything's fine. And she's ended up losing ... well it would have been twins but ... I don't know, it just makes me a bit wary and you know, like I don't know if ... there were a few questions I was going to ask today like.

(Ben: 4 yrs after diagnosis with testicular cancer)

Ben was fertile yet anxious about the impact of his testicular cancer on his sperm, but Scott had other concerns. He had not been as fortunate as some of the other men I spoke to and told me what a 'massive blow' his infertility had been:

I think in terms of where I am today, I think the biggest impact for me in what I've had to deal with, and actually quite recently, is the fact that I can't have children naturally because of all the treatment that I had. And that's actually ... probably been the biggest impact on me, and something that's taken a long, long time to actually realise. I guess once you get to your mid 30s that's the point ... and certainly my wife's at a point where you know that's either going to happen or it's not. And we've just actually been through the last couple of years a lot of procedural searches, and advice, and stuff like that through various fertility clinics, and having to see a couple of surgical procedures to look at as kind of last opportunities to find any sperm.

And that's actually been a real emotional rollercoaster in the last couple of years, because I guess in my early 20s and sort of growing up, I always felt that I would be one of the kind of lucky ones in terms of you hear about people who went through ... who are cancer survivors who went through quite a harsh regime of treatment, but they've been able to have children naturally. And I always felt that I would be one of those ... but it doesn't look as if that's going to be the case. And I'm actually currently considering all the other options. So that's ... been a massive blow.

(Scott: 18 yrs after diagnosis with acute lymphatic leukaemia)

It is significant to note Scott's reference to other men who have retained their fertility. While it is important to document the positive outcomes that in some cases defy medical prediction, there is also a danger that this can offer false hope to survivors, both male and female, whose fertility has been irreparably damaged. It may also be the case that a certain element of envy may be evoked by the success stories of others, while those who have become infertile battle with medical procedures, costly interventions and may also have to deal with failure.

Up to this point the accounts in this chapter have been from survivors who have been able to establish sexual relationships; not all of them have lasted, but there has at least been the prospect of sexual intimacy and procreation. However, we saw in the last chapter that Thomas at 30 has not had a girlfriend for 'God knows how many years', partly because of the social isolation caused by the legacy of his brain tumour. However, despite the fact that he is not currently in a relationship and does not seem optimistic about the prospect, his distress at the lack of any attempt to preserve his future ability to father a child is clear:

One of the things that I'm sad about, and didn't actually happen then, and I wasn't really aware of it, was that ... it's standard practice to take a sample of sperm or eggs from a cancer patient. Well that didn't happen ... my oncologist at the time said it wasn't necessary ... So I mean that's something one could be bitter about ... Well this chap was unfortunately a nasty bloke ... he was called Hitler as a nickname ... he was just nasty. That's another thing is that I've come across doctors who are wonderful people, and I've also come across a few who are really nasty.

(Thomas: 13 yrs after diagnosis with a brain tumour)

Thomas's account suggests that the disappointment over the prospect of infertility can be exacerbated or mitigated by the way in which it is handled by medical staff. Clearly this is a sensitive issue and if managed without care can increase distress. Thomas may have been able to avoid the bitterness he believes could have resulted from the insensitivity and lack of foresight at the time of his diagnosis and treatment, but others may not be as resilient.

Unlike Thomas, Dan is married. His relationship with his wife did not begin until their time as undergraduates was coming to an end, but because she had known him as a friend throughout the experience she knew about his testicular cancer. Despite the fact that they were now married, Dan said that he had not yet addressed the issue of fertility. When I asked him if he thought this might present any concerns in the future, he said:

> You know hopefully not. I don't think it will to be honest, because I'm quite well in myself and I think there's every chance that they will have recovered. I haven't actually made a point of not sort of checking, except for the fact that I hate the experience.
>
> (Dan: 5 yrs after diagnosis with testicular cancer)

Both Paul (unmarried) and Paul B (married), approached their uncertainty over the prospect of future fatherhood with apparent equanimity, but it was only Paul B who talked of having banked sperm:

> I guess I took the view ... I mean they did ... they explained that very clearly to me, and they explained all the options that were open. And I guess I just thought ... it wasn't my most pressing concern at the time. It's very difficult at that age to think about. When somebody's telling you have cancer and everything that comes with that word, it's very difficult to think about every ... 10 years ... it's the future I mean it's the ... you know and it doesn't ... but I guess I just thought it was one of those things that if I can I can, if I can't well then I can't and I will ... Not really. I do ... I mean I work with young people, I do like young ... and I do like, you know people with children, and I would like my own children. But if I can't have ... I know that there's plenty of children, do you know what I mean?
>
> (Paul: 9 yrs after diagnosis with testicular cancer)

I can't have children. We were considering it, going looking at obviously the ... what do you call it? [sperm banking] So yes, I mean that's something we would consider in a few years maybe. I fill in the forms to keep them all stored and everything, but that's it for the time being. I mean we do obviously think about it, but we've sort of planned it maybe in the next few years, if we decide to. At the moment we're just not in a position to ... but as I say we're keeping them all, everything stored up. So it's ... we have it there if in the future we decide so it's good.

> (Paul B: 11 yrs after diagnosis with non-Hodgkin's lymphoma)

Jack had been too ill to bank sperm before his treatment and though, 'just in case' his fertility was unimpaired, he and his girlfriend had been using contraception, he had recently undergone a fertility test which had confirmed his infertility.

> The treatment made me infertile as well, which is another thing. And I find in a way that's … that's like another physical repercussion … I mean it's changed in all ways – you know physically, mentally, possibly emotionally as well. And I found that hard to talk about certainly in my teens when I knew about it, but now I just think you know it's certainly not a thing to be ashamed of.
>
> (Jack: 9 yrs after diagnosis with Hodgkin's lymphoma)

John, speaking about his inability to father a child, more than 30 years after diagnosis, said that at that time there was no preparation for the prospect of infertility and no options such as sperm banking were offered. However, he and his wife had, after many difficulties, succeeded in adopting two children:

> Because of the treatment I couldn't have any family. That was never broached by the medical establishment … it wasn't until, you know I'd been married over 12 month[s], nothing of course was happening. And went to see the GP who sat and squirmed in his seat, and clearly there was something amiss. And he said because of the treatment you won't have any family … there was no sperm banking back in the 70s – certainly not in the North East anyway. But of course that brought new dilemmas, and also new challenges, because we approached a number of adoption agencies, who again didn't want to know us because of my past history, because adoptive agencies can be so selective with parents. They didn't want to know me because of my cancer history. We even went down to Sheffield teaching hospital to try and be accepted for artificial insemination, and again the approach was that you know I was too much of a risk, and that they didn't advocate single-parent families … eventually we fostered a little girl with a view to long-term adoption, and that proved very fruitful.
>
> (John: 33 yrs after diagnosis with Hodgkin's lymphoma)

While John's account of the lack of preparation for infertility might be thought to have been an outdated phenomenon, Michael too, only 5 years after diagnosis, said that his future fertility had not been mentioned as an issue but he had read about the possible implications:

> From what I've read sort of in the build up to having the treatments and things, you know I was doing a lot of reading on books, and sort of picked up on the fact that when I was younger I had a hernia and an undescended testes, and obviously testicular cancer as well. So, all those

things tend to lead me to believe that I'm likely to be less fertile than a normal guy. But I've not crossed that bridge yet.

(Michael: 5 yrs after diagnosis with testicular cancer)

Summary

All the interview material used in this chapter suggests strongly that the impact on fertility, or concerns about the impact on fertility continue to have repercussions for many years. There is no doubt that this effect is life stage related and of particular relevance to those who were diagnosed when young adults. Whether their concerns relate to a perceived lack of support and information, as shown in Vicky's account, or whether they manifest as anxiety for the health of children conceived successfully, uncertainty and anxiety can result. Lesley even worried for her daughter's future fertility and the health of potential grandchildren could also be a concern.

There seems to be evidence of a patchy service at the time of diagnosis both in terms of the provision of information and of the availability of options for the preservation of fertility. It is also the case that some participants who were warned at the time that they would become infertile were not infertile, and some who had not been warned about the risk discovered that they were infertile. It may be impossible to state with any certainty at the time of diagnosis and treatment what the outcome for fertility will be, but we can see that life plans are made on the basis of what survivors may believe to be factual medical information. In some cases where this has presented an unexpected outcome, the effects have been far-reaching. The patchiness of the information and opportunities for fertility preservation at the time of the illness evident in the earlier accounts, appear to support the assertions made by Schover (2007), Shaw *et al.* (2004) and Reebals *et al.* (2006) discussed at the start of this chapter. However, what we can chart from the interviews is the enormity of the impact across many years.

Even those who had remained unconcerned about fertility at the time of their diagnosis later experienced some anxiety. Indeed, because of their age at diagnosis it may only be some time after recovery that the enormity of the impact is realised and when this happens it may not be obvious where to turn for help. We saw in Chapter 4 that there is a need for some kind of ongoing support and for a continuing source of information after long-term follow-up has ended. It seems that such a need also exists in relation to advice over fertility. However, when planning such services it is also important to remember that the hospital environment can be experienced as intimidating and reminiscent of past distress and further medical intervention can carry an emotional and negative meaning for cancer survivors. While this might be a price most survivors are willing to pay for a successful outcome in their attempt to become parents, those health professionals who are treating survivors need to be aware that it is not only their cancer history that may be relevant, but also the emotional legacy of their illness.

The provision of accessible and timely information may be crucial, particularly for female survivors. Several of my female participants told me that they had been advised that they should not attempt to conceive within 5 years of treatment lest it increase the likelihood of a recurrence of their cancer. Yet some had not been aware that they would also be at risk from an early menopause. Clearly under such circumstances the window of opportunity for conception may be small. This could be a particular problem for the age group who might not – because of their life stage – be in relationships which would lead to pregnancy.

Clearly not all survivors are able to retain their fertility, and the proportion of my participants who have conceived without medical intervention may not be representative of survivors in general. For those who do require medical intervention it seems that there are some practitioners who are less than sensitive to their needs, physical, emotional and financial. We have already seen that the legacy of the illness can have a lasting financial impact, and for survivors to be confronted with the options presented to Mary seems to denote a lack of understanding of the effect that cancer in this age group has on all aspects of life – even years after the event.

Acknowledging that this is an extremely sensitive issue, Schover (2007: 264) suggests that 'psychosocial counselling and education may increase the efficacy of purely physiological interventions'. This appears to be an eminently sensible proposition; however, I encountered no evidence of such provision from my participants. But as Schover goes on to argue, there has been very little evidence-based knowledge available for the guidance of oncologists 'in remediating reproductive health issues'. I hope that this chapter will contribute to an understanding of the issue as it is experienced by young men and women who face a childless or uncertain reproductive future.

Key points

* Information on fertility for both men and women at the point of diagnosis is patchy
* The option of fertility preservation techniques is not always apparent or possible
* Lack of concern over fertility at the time of diagnosis can be followed by regret in later years
* A great deal of emotional distress is caused by not knowing where to go for fertility advice after treatment
* For those men and women whose fertility had been proven, concerns over their children's health can ensue
* Unfounded assumptions about fertility or infertility can affect relationships and result in their failure
* Ongoing support relating to fertility issues, both practical and emotional, would benefit many long-term survivors
* The providers of such support need to be aware of the emotional legacy of the cancer as well as the physical effects

9 Implications for policy and practice

The accounts on which this volume is based are drawn from survivors whose only common experience is that they had cancer as adolescents, young adults. All other contextual details and life events represent a wide range of social, educational and economic circumstances, marital status, ages, gender and duration of survivorship. As Soliman and Agresta (2008: 59) say many factors including age, personality, faith, education, culture, family, social support, financial means, prognosis and quality of life can shape the ability to deal with the challenges of survivorship. Yet, despite the heterogeneity of my participants, it has been possible to identify a commonality of experience and identification of issues that has allowed the interview data to be presented thematically.

There are, of course, some contrasting experiences that have been commented on throughout the empirical chapters, but even here there is an overlap in the identification of significant issues. It is perhaps the similarity between accounts from such disparate participants that is the most surprising element of the interview data. For example the striking likeness between the positive statements at the end of Chapter 5 and other examples of almost verbatim repetition in the way the experiences and feelings about survivorship are described and discussed.

Yet there is also dissonance – how is it possible for such consistently positive interpretations to be made, as quoted in Chapter 5, when other chapters have contained accounts of pain, distress, anxiety and disruption to life plans? Have I selectively drawn from accounts that have no bearing on each other? The book is not organised around individual narratives in a linear fashion, thus it is difficult to follow through a single participant's story, but were this to be done it would be apparent that there are internal contradictions and inconsistencies even in one person's narrative. The experience of long-term survivorship is not constant, nor is it linear. Events can catapult a survivor back into a state resembling PTS, yet the same person may feel that their perspective on life has been enhanced by the cancer experience. Life chances can open up positive opportunities directly related to the cancer, but equally options can be closed down by the same illness history. Some of the 'late effects' that are attributed to the cancer may have been experienced in any case, but it is of significance that the cancer is central to their explanation – even many years later. In addition, survivorship identity – public or private – carried through life may shape later interactions and relationships, both personal and professional.

Langeveld and Arbuckle (2008) argue that long-term survivors are increasing in both number and age and that this carries with it a need for health care services to develop appropriate expertise and resources to meet their needs. Langeveld and Arbuckle offer a model of what provision should look like to achieve successful transition from paediatric to adult services, but this addresses only one dimension of survivorship and only at a particular moment in time. The testimonies in this volume point to a life-long survivorship effect that includes physical, emotional and social dimensions. The concomitant requirements for appropriate support are extremely complex with different needs being manifested at different stages.

While the accounts of treatments experienced many years earlier may now be dated, the evidence from all the participants who contributed to this study suggests strongly that survivorship after cancer in adolescence and young adulthood carries with it life-long implications and that there is an attendant need for some form of continuing support to be made available. Langeveld and Arbuckle acknowledge this and say that there is a need to develop 'a systematic plan for health care that extends not just through childhood and adolescence, but also through the lifetime of the survivor' (2008: 160–161). However, according to these authors, while the need for long-term surveillance is clear, what has been less clear is how it should be designed. Earle *et al.* (2007: 287) suggest that many cancer survivors are 'lost in transition' and that the quality of care suffers because neither patients nor providers know what should be expected at the end of treatment.

I hope that the testimonies in this volume offer some insight into the continuing and changing needs of survivors. Based on the evidence gathered from the participants, the remainder of this volume considers what factors need to be understood and how they influence the provision of appropriate ongoing care and support for life-long survivorship.

Preparation for late effects

Many of the accounts in this book suggest that some participants were not well prepared for the long-term impact the cancer would have on their lives. Those who were relating accounts from many years earlier may not be representative of the 'open awareness' (Field 2002) context that supposedly prevails currently. However, there was evidence that some of those treated more recently had felt confused about what to expect in the longer-term, while some participants who had been treated decades earlier had, in fact, been well prepared. This suggests a patchiness of experience and a lack of consistency across treatment centres. However, what the contrasting accounts expose is that honesty at the time of diagnosis was important and that this approach established a trusting relationship, not only with the health professionals caring for them at the time, but that this was extended to those who would care for them in the future. While professionals might have concerns at the point of diagnosis that a bleak outlook and warnings of all the possible long-term consequences would be more than the patient could cope with, a gradual sharing of information delivered in an *age-appropriate* way (Grinyer 2007) was thought to be the best means of preparation. A positive interpretation at the time – whatever the prognosis – appeared to act as a lens through which to view the illness in a way that was lasting and shaped future encounters with health professionals.

The late effects of the cancer and its treatment may change as time progresses, and there will be occasions, for example, like the realisation that mantle field radiotherapy can increase the risk of breast cancer – when survivors need to be recalled for screening. Of course an event such as this will not, by definition, have been predicted at the time of treatment, yet there is evidence in the testimonies in this book that the way in which such recalls are dealt with can have far-reaching emotional effects as well as a possible impact on the medical outcome. Recalls can be mismanaged or – even worse – not made at all and the survivor may discover via the Internet or other media that they could be at risk. Under such circumstances they at least need to know that their GP is aware of the problem, has kept up to date with the latest knowledge on late effects and treatments and is willing to refer as appropriate. The next section addresses long-term follow-up after official clinic appointments have terminated, suffice it to say that if a positive relationship, perceived as supportive, has been established with a particular clinic where the patient is known, there may be a reduction in the traumatic impact associated with such recalls and any subsequent tests. Even though over time staff may change there should be a degree of continuity that is reassuring.

A central aspect of preparation for late effects relates to fertility for both males and females. While it may be accepted practice to advise the young adult at the time of diagnosis that either the illness or the treatment may affect their fertility, the implications are not always clear as they may be lost on a young person who might never have considered parenthood and for whom infertility seems a remote and distant effect. Many of the survivors will wish to become parents and even if they have been prepared during their treatment for the challenges that can arise in relation to fertility, easily accessible advice should be forthcoming throughout their survivorship. This should extend to pre and post natal care both of which can be affected by their previous illness and treatment history. We have seen an account in this volume of a case where the implications did not appear to be well understood by those offering maternity care and where the survivor's health was compromised as a result. Again this suggests a lack of continuity and communication between centres and specialisms that can leave the survivor feeling that, because a cancer history at this age is rare, the implications are not always well understood in obstetric and maternity services.

Some survivors have found it difficult to access ongoing support and advice on reproductive matters. Such provision could be made available on a needs basis so that, at a time chosen by the survivor, access to fertility expertise and whatever tests are deemed appropriate, is easily negotiated. While such a service may already be in place after treatment in age-specific facilities, the accounts in this volume suggest that this provision is not universal and information can be difficult to access. It is also the case that to support the medical input, counselling may be helpful in supporting the survivor emotionally through what may be experienced as a challenging process.

Follow-up clinics

In relation to the clinical aspects, Langeveld and Arbuckle (2008) say, the success of any long-term follow-up programme is dependent on participation by the survivors who will have views on their needs. While some of the suggestions for support made thus far may be appropriately delivered in late effects or long-term follow-up clinics, there was much evidence that the experience of long-term follow-up can be a difficult process. Careful thought should be given to how the clinics are organised, where they are held and in what context – for example, the integration of those in long-term follow-up with patients in active receipt of treatment can result in the distressing recall of the treatment experience. This may appear to be 'stating the obvious' yet during informal discussions with staff in follow-up clinics it became clear that under the pressure of clinic schedules, for staff a satisfactory consultation is one in which the patient materialises and their results are clear. The anxiety that may have preceded and accompanied that visit, and the impact of the clinic environment, remain largely unobserved by staff and unarticulated by patients.

Feuerstein comments on the lack of awareness amongst survivors that the 'quarterly ritual' of follow-up clinics, which causes so much anticipatory anxiety, can be alleviated with appropriate medications or self-management strategies (2007: 483). He asks why physicians do not routinely offer such options. Yet if the health professionals remain unaware of the meaning of the clinic and, as I suggest, are concerned primarily with monitoring for recurrence, such a strategy may not occur to them.

When the final clinic visit has been made, relief can be swiftly followed by panic at the thought of being cut adrift from support and medical scrutiny. As a result some streamlined access to expert advice without having to be referred via a GP may be valued. For example, a website with 'Frequently Asked Questions' might be accompanied by a telephone advice line that takes callers through to a professional who can access their records, who knows their case history and who can refer them to an appropriate consultant for an appointment if necessary. Such provision could meet many of the needs expressed by participants.

Carol, a Macmillan nurse, makes some suggestions as to how ongoing support might be delivered and recognises the need for flexibility in a system that may often be administered in an inflexible and bureaucratic manner:

> I definitely think that's a role for specialist nurses ... people ... often relate better to a nurse than to doctors. I do nurse-led follow-up clinics ... very often there's a set protocol for how long people will be followed up which is only 3 years. Now for some people ... they feel afraid of being cast adrift ... I have autonomy over those clinics ... so I don't actually discharge them at 3 years but offer them the choice of whether they want to be discharged or if they prefer to keep coming back to see me ... we have half-hour appointments for each person and because it's always me that they see, it's not random other people, we know each other ... they really do seem to appreciate that ... in between [appointments] if they have any concerns then they ring up and I'll see them sooner to address that concern. And then if necessary I'd arrange an appointment with one of the consultants. And it's done so much more quickly then, than going through the GP.
>
> (Carol: Macmillan nurse)

Of course one of the characteristics of the age group around the time of diagnosis and treatment is that they are likely to move away geographically from their place of care as they embark on further education, seek employment or marry, thus they may not have access to the continuity of care and support suggested by Carol earlier. Under such circumstances an easily identifiable transitional pathway that would enable their case to be passed on to another centre would be necessary. Again such provision may already exist in some places, but there are enough intimations of a lack of communication and smooth transfer in this volume to suggest that the service can be patchy.

The testimonies in this volume show that the needs of survivors can continue beyond the follow-up phase and extend into later life even decades after diagnosis and treatment. Yet even survivors who may have the option of continuing clinical follow-up for life may not wish to attend clinics. This as we have seen can carry with it an emotional legacy that acts as a reminder of their potential vulnerability and status as a cancer patient. If this is the case, alternative strategies need to be adopted to meet those ongoing needs; it is to these options that we now turn.

Ongoing support: meeting emotional and psychological needs

In addition to the need for easily accessible medical advice, there may also be a role for a less formal support network. Based on extensive knowledge of survivorship issues expressed by the people who seek information and support from his telephone helpline, Ashley, a participant who is quoted throughout this volume, suggests that support groups can play a central role in survivors' lives and has strong views about how this can best be provided:

> I think [support] can best come from fellow sufferers ... many ... charities have support groups up and down the country that meet on a regular basis ... they make themselves a cup of tea and have a few biscuits but the main reason that they're doing it is to compare notes, and to be aware of the fact that they're not alone, that there are other people out there in the same boat as them, who have had the [same] experiences as them. Because the feeling that you are alone with this, and handling it on your own, and even your friends and family who don't have this diagnosis, no matter how well meaning they are, and how caring and loving they are, they don't know what it's like. So being with fellow sufferers, even if it's only at the end of the phone, and being able to talk to people ... And that's wonderful. It really is wonderful. And I've spoken to people who've gone along to support groups for the first time, and having had a diagnosis for like 20 or 30 years, and they ring me up, and their life has been changed by it.
>
> (Ashley: 37 yrs after diagnosis with CTCL)

However, while there may be some excellent support services run by the voluntary or charitable sectors, discussions with professionals who recommend them suggest that they may not be acceptable or feel accessible to some who regard them as very 'middle class'. As Carol observed with regards to a patient:

> She went once and she said, 'I'm not going there again.' She lived on a council estate, she said, 'I'm not going there again. They're all too snobby up there' ... I mean they're very good, the services that they provide ... but it was [not] her [culture].
>
> (Carol: Macmillan nurse)

These two well-informed comments from Ashley and Carol – one a survivor whose life's work has been determined by his illness and the other a health professional who sees a range of survivors – demonstrate that 'one size does not fit all'. Indeed this is also clear from the participants, not all of whom would have welcomed what they perceived to be 'ghettoisation', and for whom support groups would not be experienced as helpful. Thus, ideally, there should be different support options that would be acceptable to people with a variety of possibly changing needs who are also from different social contexts.

It is clear from the way in which participants spoke of the ongoing emotional impact on their lives – even many years after the illness – that there may also be a need for some input from professional health care services This may be required only sporadically, but as and when it is necessary it should be easy to access, non stigmatised and appropriate to their stage of survivorship. That this need is currently unmet for many was articulated not only by the participants but also in the following extract from an interview with Carol, a health professional, who suggests that men in particular may have problems in acknowledging need and accessing services:

> Where the national ... cancer treatment falls down, is the lack of psychological services ... .it can be difficult for some people to say 'yes I do want some help'. But if it's seen as ... just part of the treatment this is part of your care, and it's a norm ... that misperception that people have that in seeking psychological services and support, that they're weak, because it's not weak ... I think there should be different kinds ... [of] psychological support for men, or boys ... if we take out the word therapy, then men might participate a little bit more ... I think we need to look at different ways of dealing [with young men] things like having a five-a-side football match or something. You know something, having some kind of forum which isn't seen as health care if you like, or psychological services but could be run by good psychologists or therapists.
>
> (Carol: Macmillan nurse)

Inhibiting factors may be gender related as suggested by Carol who said of support groups: 'young men: there's no way that they'll be going there.' Based on this assumption, Carol suggested the possible need for a lateral approach to support being more likely to succeed with men. However, despite Carol's assumption that men would need the 'lateral football approach' – which indeed may be appropriate in some situations – I found no consistent difference in gender-related needs, there were as many women who would resist belonging to a support group as there were men who thought it might help.

Across the gender divide, to some extent the differential between those who expressed a need for support and those who did not was explained by the presence – or absence – of a strong family or social network. As I discovered in my research on the impact on families (Grinyer 2002a) and my interviews with young people in treatment (2007) families are of central importance at the time of the illness, but their role in supporting the survivor continues well after the treatment period is over. For those survivors who were well supported socially there appeared to be less need for any emotional support to be organised formally. Access to such personal support structures will of course change over time, particularly in this age group as the young person moves away from home and separates from dependence on family (Grinyer 2002a). As a result, the need to be able to move in and out of formal support structures may be of significant importance as life circumstances change.

So it seems that survivors need to be listened to carefully and no assumptions made about what they would find acceptable or unacceptable. While some would like to belong to a support group of peers; others would like to offer their experience in support of such a group. Some participants were very resistant to the notion of being 'ghettoised' while other survivors were more amenable to the notion of a social grouping with those of a similar age. For those who would find a support group helpful it is important to bear in mind the meaning that the hospital environment has for survivors and to locate the group in a more neutral setting that does not necessitate a return to a medical environment, in particular the place of care, which can hold so many painful and traumatic memories.

Resource and Policy Implications

Soliman and Agresta (2008) say that a concerted effort is needed to increase funding for additional research to improve survivorship outcomes. Hopefully this study has contributed towards the knowledge necessary to develop services that will meet the needs expressed in this volume. But what might appropriate provision look like and what are the resource implications? Is a 'critical mass' necessary before it is feasible to offer a support service? Feuerstein argues the case for innovative services that are offered consistently over the long term for survivors and says the following:

> These services need to be better structured to facilitate access, provide unique modes of delivery and services, and provide these services in sites other than tertiary medical centres (e.g. community-based clinics) … There is a need for better understanding and effective approaches that smoothly reintegrate the cancer survivor into society.
>
> (Feuerstein 2007: 487)

Feuerstein emphasises the difficulties that can be experienced in reintegration into the workplace – clearly a potential problem for all cancer survivors but for those whose career is at its very beginnings, this may present an even greater challenge. This author also suggests that there is a need for more education and training on the complexities of cancer survivorship and its management. It is important to remember that Feuerstein is referring to cancer survivors in general rather than to a specific age group. Yet, if there is a paucity of knowledge relating to survivorship in general, the chances are that there is an even greater knowledge gap surrounding the needs of survivors of adolescent and young adult cancers who, as we have seen, experience distinct age and life stage related challenges that are not well documented.

According to Feuerstein, survivors would benefit from being trained in self-management skills. Such skills would assist in the ability to take greater control over health care and other issues that impact on the quality of life. Again this author is referring to all age groups, and again we can see that such provision may be particularly necessary and beneficial for the survivors of adolescent cancers whose self-management strategies may not have had an opportunity to be well developed prior to the illness.

A summary of the USA's Institute of Medicine's (IOM) recommendation provides some indication of the benefits of a 'survivorship care plan':

- Primary care physicians need to be more aware of survivorship issues.
- Primary care physicians should have access to details of prior treatments and diagnosis via the survivorship care plan.
- Guidelines on optimal survivorship care are needed and could be supported by Randomised Controlled Trials (RCT) in survivorship care.
- Collaboration is needed between primary care physicians and cancer specialists – a shared care model can merge resources and talents.
- A common understanding between specialist and primary carers, the easy transfer of records and seamless handovers should help to mitigate the disruption caused by fragmented care.
- The management of other complex conditions (such as heart disease, diabetes, AIDS, IBS and Parkinson's) shared between primary and specialist physicians could be used as a model of best practice.

(adapted from Earle *et al.* 2007: 291–292)

As Feuerstein (2007) says the implementation of such a plan would improve knowledge and communication among providers and between providers and survivors which could only benefit any survivor of cancer in whatever age bracket. However, while the suggestions in this plan may offer potential benefits through enhanced services, they are all focused on improving the liaison between primary and tertiary services. While such measures should be welcomed, the testimonies in this volume speak of additional, and largely unmet, emotional and social needs.

The UK's Cancer Reform Strategy (Department of Health 2007) recognises the need to support survivors of cancer and contains a section on a National Cancer Survivorship Initiative to take this part of the strategy forward in partnership with Macmillan Cancer Support. There is recognition that such an initiative requires collaboration between primary and secondary care physicians, social care services, service users, patients and the voluntary sector. The following approaches may be used to support survivors:

- Clinical follow-up by hospital doctors, nurses and/or GPs to monitor late effects
- Education, self care and expert patient programmes
- Proactive case management e.g. by telephone
- Drop-in centres for peer support
- Automated surveillance systems to ensure appropriate testing
- Patient reports using electronic means such as mobile phones
- Rehabilitation programmes
- Psychological and spiritual support
- Back-to-work support

- Access to financial and benefits advice
- Nutritional advice
  (adapted from Department of Health *Cancer Reform Strategy* 2007: 81)

A commentary on this list does acknowledge that there should be a consideration of how these strategies can be tailored to meet individual patients' needs; and this could include a consideration of survivors of cancer in adolescence and young adulthood as a distinct group. The document as a whole does contain a section on age-appropriate services and mentions the TCT wards and the importance of age-specific treatment centres. Thus it is to be hoped that there will be an associated recognition that survivors of cancer in this age group are likely to need a tailored approach to their continued support.

It would be unrealistic not to take into account the other illness and patient groups all competing for limited funds as clearly the provision of additional services would have cost and resource implications. However, despite the attendant funding requirements, the longer-term outcomes may offset any additional expense. We have seen the level of need amongst the survivors, who being at the start of their productive adult lives have the potential to contribute much to wider society for many years. However, they also have the potential to be users of large amounts of resources for an extended period should they experience continuing psychological or physical ill health. Thus a strategy to mitigate any detrimental effects after cancer is to be welcomed – even at an initial set-up cost.

Discussing the cost-consequences of surveillance, Earle claims the only outcome of any real importance is an increase in the quantity and/or quality of life (2007: 50). However, to gain the backing for improving provision for survivors, as Feuerstein (2007) argues, there is a need for society to view the problems of cancer survivors as a genuine health concern. I would add to this that there also needs to be recognition that survivors in different age categories need tailored services and this too should be recognised as a public health concern.

While this volume has focused on survivorship after adolescent and young adult cancer, I wish to reiterate my comment in Chapter 1 that in no sense do I intend to diminish the difficulties experienced by survivors in other age categories. Indeed while my suggestions for provision are based on the age-specific focus of my study, I hope that some of my findings and recommendations might also be of wider applicability and that those who fall outside the adolescent and young adult cancer survivor category may benefit from improving our understanding and knowledge of survivorship and the challenges that survivors face.

Finally ...

The purpose of this book was to understand the long-term implications after cancer in adolescence and young adulthood, not primarily to establish that life stage at diagnosis continues to have consequences for the survivor. Nevertheless, while there is no doubt that a long-term effect is widely experienced, and that those experiences have much in common, it also became apparent that the life stage impact does in many instances permeate long-term survivorship in the same way that it affects the period around diagnosis and treatment.

The lasting impact on fertility – whether it is preserved or not – shapes choices that other young adults do not have to make. That education is not yet completed and careers may not yet have begun or been established fully at the point of diagnosis – has a lasting effect on life plans and on finances. The social impact continues to be felt for the same reason – the illness separates young adults from their peers at a crucial transitional stage that can continue to affect activities and relationships long into recovery. The emotional impact of all these can also permeate decades of survivorship.

Identities not yet formed fully can also be shaped by the illness; a life-changing experience at this critical moment in life can determine not only how the young people perceive themselves but also how they relate to the world and define their role within it. And if adolescence and young adulthood is a critical time for the shaping of destinies it is also a moment in time when the philosophy of life can be determined.

The distinct needs of adolescents and young adults with cancer – medical, psychological, social and educational, have been researched and established as requiring age-appropriate provision (Albritton and Bleyer 2003, Arbuckle *et al.* 2005, Grinyer 2007, Morgan and Hubber 2004). On the basis of the evidence in this volume, gathered from participants at all stages of long-term survivorship, I would argue that survivors of adolescent and young adult cancer require similar recognition as a group who experience particular challenges and whose survival is to some extent shaped by their age at diagnosis. This volume has presented the verbatim voices of survivors in a bid to communicate what is particular and distinctive about their survivorship. I hope that the power of their testimony has made the case for their needs to be recognised and met.

While many of the effects discussed in this volume could be defined as 'negative', I want the final words in this book to reflect the positivity and courage that permeates the participants' testimonies and to quote Kelly who said 'I wouldn't take it back for a million pounds'.

Appendix

Methods

Data were collected from participants located in two National Health Service (NHS) hospital Trusts, from participants recruited through two charities and through an informal network by recommendation and word of mouth. A list of participants including their age, illness type and their age at diagnosis is included at the beginning of this volume. Access and recruitment procedures varied in all locations and are discussed later. The data were collected through qualitative interviews that adopted a grounded theory approach (Glaser and Strauss 1967). Thus as new issues were raised by participants they were fed into subsequent interviews. However, I also gave the participants the opportunity to discuss their experience in an unstructured way thus ensuring that issues of significance to them had a chance of being raised.

In the first Trust eligible patients were identified by the Oncology Outpatient Clinic sister. The inclusion and exclusion criteria as agreed upon by the NHS Ethics Committee were clear. The patient should have been diagnosed with their cancer between the ages of 14–25 and should be at least 5 years out of treatment at the time of the interview. As the clinic was a general outpatients' clinic, the majority of patients were not eligible either in terms of their age at diagnosis or their stage of treatment. Indeed many of the patients at the clinic were attending in order to have treatment. Thus the proportion of attendees at any given clinic eligible for recruitment was minimal.

On a number of occasions I travelled to the clinic having been alerted by staff that several patients who fulfilled the inclusion criteria had appointments for that day. However, as became clear through interviews that I did manage to conduct, there was a degree of ambivalence about attendance. This was not a clinic specifically for long-term follow-up patients. As such, the atmosphere, in the presence of other patients who were being treated, was found to be challenging. I was not informed of the non-attendance rate for the clinic as a whole, but for my cohort it appeared to be high. The potential participants were largely young men who had been diagnosed with testicular cancer – not a demographic whose characteristics include the seeking of medical advice. On one occasion, I had travelled to the clinic with the prospect of four eligible participants attending for their appointments – not one of them materialised. As a result recruitment was slow. It is tempting to attribute cause to low attendance, however without the opportunity to interview the non-attenders I can only speculate and extrapolate from those I did interview.

Potential participants were identified by a staff member and introduced to me. If the system had been working well they should have had a patient information sheet in the post the previous week to alert them to the possibility of being asked to contribute, but this was not always the case. All patients approached at the clinic agreed to be interviewed, apart from one who wished to consider participation and asked me to telephone him the following week. When I called him as arranged he declined an interview without giving any reason. Ultimately, despite visiting this clinic at regular intervals over a number of months I carried out only eight interviews.

The interviews with patients at this clinic were not easy to conduct. In accordance with the protocol, I gave the prospective participants the option of how, when and where to be interviewed. I offered them the chance to think it over and be interviewed at a later date at a location of their choice; to be interviewed later by telephone or to find a 'quiet' location and to be interviewed while awaiting their appointment or straight afterward. The majority elected to be interviewed 'on the spot' and did not seem to be concerned if this was semi-public in the waiting room or cafeteria. However, the background noise and my consciousness of potential breaches of confidentiality did not always make this an easy option. Nevertheless, I was always led by the participants' preference.

The second Trust to allow me access to their patients did so in a very ad hoc way. Largely through personal recollection, a list of eligible ex patients was drawn up. The length of the list (approximately 12) was promising, but all those on it needed to be contacted initially by a staff member, in the end only three people on the list were referred to me. I interviewed them in their homes at their suggestion. However, personal contact with a staff member at the Breast Clinic in the same Trust revealed a potential source of eligible patients as some of the women attendees were having follow-up checks after adolescent lymphoma. This source of patients led to five interviews. Interestingly one of these patients, who had been treated for lymphoma 14 years earlier and was a member of the Lymphoma Association, suggested that the Association might be willing to put me in touch with other members. Thus in a variation of snowball sampling a rich seam of participants was generated.

The Lymphoma Association agreed to post an appeal for participants on their website and in their newsletter. This approach resulted in 14 interviews undertaken over the telephone. Participants were self selected and some did not match the exact inclusion criteria of age at diagnosis. However I felt that it was important to let them tell their stories. There is always something to be learned from hearing people's accounts – even if it relates to the difference between those diagnosed and treated at a particular age and those younger or older. But more importantly if someone has taken the trouble to respond to an appeal for research participants, particularly when the topic is of such personal and potentially painful concern, I believe that the right thing to do is to listen to them.

It could be argued that the recruitment of participants from a disease-specific association would skew the data towards a particular illness. However, lymphoma is a cancer frequently diagnosed in adolescence and young adulthood, and the other sites of recruitment tended to specialise in germ cell tumours or sarcomas, thus to some extent the balance was redressed. The spread of cancer types amongst the participants represents a wide range of illnesses though some cancers, such as brain tumours, are underrepresented, but this may be a function of the likelihood of long-term survivorship and the degree of debility experienced in the aftermath.

An additional source of recruitment was through the Teenage Cancer Trust (TCT). A member of the senior management used his personal knowledge of a number of long-term survivors in order to recruit for me and this resulted in a further eight interviews. The participants recruited from both the TCT and the Lymphoma Association were interviewed by telephone as they were scattered across the country and the project did not have the resources to allow for travel to each location (Thomas and Purdon 1994). However, I was unable to discern any substantial impact on the quality of the resulting interview data which were rich and detailed, the phone conversations usually lasting for at least as long as any of the face-to-face interviews. In some cases it may even have been preferable to use the telephone as a medium as participants were able to address sensitive issues about sexuality and body image that could for some present greater difficulties in person. While these two sources of participants had not been part of the original research design, they were in the end essential to its success or sufficient numbers would not have been generated. Finally, a number of participants were recruited through informal contacts and recommendations, this source generated 11 interviews.

Interviews lasted from between 20 minutes to an hour and a half. The shorter interviews tended to be with young men and the lengthier ones with the older participants both male and female. The location of the interview did not appear to have a direct effect on the duration as some of the longer ones took place on hospital premises and the telephone interviews were also some of the longer ones. While greater detail and depth was achieved through the longer interviews, the shorter ones still provided some interesting information on the experience of survivorship.

All participants were offered the chance to select a pseudonym, but most preferred that their own first names be used. The use of real names can appear to be in contravention of codes of ethical conduct and I have written on this topic elsewhere (Grinyer 2002b). However, as my approach with the participants in all aspects of the conduct of this study was that they should lead the process, I respected their wish to retain 'ownership' of their stories through the use of their real names if they wished. All interviews were recorded with consent and subsequently transcribed verbatim.

Sampling was not possible as all participants, apart from those who contacted me directly, were approached and recruited by an intermediary, thus the sample was to some extent a convenience one of those who happened to be attending the clinic on a particular day, or were recalled by staff in an ad hoc way as being eligible. Despite this process, over which I had little control, the range of ages, illnesses, life circumstances, lengths of time since diagnosis and treatment, and the gender distribution suggest that a relevant range of characteristics have been captured in the sample.

Data were collected until saturation had been reached. Glaser and Strauss (1967) refer to this process as 'theoretical saturation', which refers to the point at which observations no longer serve to question or modify theories generated from earlier data (May 1997: 144). In order to make such a judgement, the collection of qualitative data incorporates a process of ongoing analysis throughout the data collection period (Robson 1995). When new issues are raised by a participant these can be taken out into subsequent interviews, thus while the topics have been generated by the interviewees in the first instance, the researcher can use them as the basis of a topic guide for future interviews.

While the researcher is constantly developing an analytical framework throughout the process, it is nevertheless crucial that analytical transparency and rigour are demonstrated if qualitative data are to avoid being dismissed as 'merely anecdotal' or highly selective. Mindful of such a requirement, the data were rigorously analysed using methods of data reduction, display and conclusion drawing (Miles and Huberman 1994). Miles and Huberman (1994) note that extended text is dispersed, poorly structured and extremely bulky, and that in order to avoid jumping to unfounded conclusions, or overweighting a particularly dramatic passage, certain processes must be observed during analysis. To this end the data have been subjected to codification. They have been sorted and sifted in a manner that facilitates the identification of similar phrases, themes and patterns. Through the identification of commonalties and differences, and a consideration of the relationship between the variables, a set of generalisations was gradually developed to cover the consistencies discerned in the database.

Ethics

The research was of course approved through an NHS Ethics Committee. However, the problems with recruitment through the NHS and the consequent need to approach potential participants through alternative routes necessitated additional ethical approval for this approach, this was granted by my University's Ethics Committee. Of central concern in my application was of the protection of participants from harm. As such certain safeguards were built into the research design. Provision for their support was on hand should they become distressed, they could stop the interview at any time and could withdraw their data at a later stage if they wished. All had a patient

information sheet with details of the research and ways in wish to contact me
should they wish to do so.

Only one participant became emotional during the course of the interview
undertaken in the hospital café after his annual outpatient appointment. I
offered to turn the tape off and end the interview but he said that he wished
to continue. Concerned that he might have felt distressed in the aftermath I
offered to arrange for him to get support from a staff member. He declined
the offer and said the following:

> It's like it was nice to be asked about your … I think that's one of the most
> important. That's something which could be done, to be asked … to be
> asked about what your experience has been.
>
> (Paul: 9 yrs after diagnosis with testicular cancer)

Paul's emotional reaction and response to my concern suggest that while
engagement in research that requires the recollection of painful or distressing
memories can be difficult and emotional, this does not mean that it does not
have a value for the participant. My follow-up study of the parents of young
adults with cancer (most of whom had died) spoke of the cathartic and ther-
apeutic effects of participation. Despite an acknowledgement of the emotional demands of participation, the perceived validation and legitimation of
their experience more than compensated (Grinyer 2004). As Linda, one of the
participants included in this volume said: 'I am grateful for the conversation'
and this type of comment was not unusual at the end of interviews when I
asked if the participant would like to say anything else. Even Linda who I
interviewed 28 years after her cancer diagnosis, during which time she had
spoken to few people about her experience, addressed distressing events that
could have been construed as intrusive and painful, yet appeared to value the
opportunity to discuss her cancer and its aftermath.

Summary

The data drawn upon so heavily in this volume are, I believe, its strength.
There are verbatim extracts of first-hand experiences that, while organised
into themed chapters, nevertheless allow the participants' voices to be heard.
The accounts come from a variety of sources, across a range of individuals
who had been diagnosed with a variety of cancers at differing lengths of time
since their original diagnosis, the shortest being 4 years and the longest 48
years. The participants came not only through NHS sites, but also through
charitable organisations, by word of mouth and through the informal
network of those whose families had been involved in the first phase of the
research with parents of young adults with cancer.

The difficulties of access meant that this was a hard group to reach; they
tended not to congregate together. Indeed they may have nothing in common
other than their cancer survivorship – their ages ranged from early 20s to

early 60s and they came from all parts of the British Isles. These factors resulted in recruitment being slow and the accumulation of the eventual cohort took over a year. It was proved necessary to adapt the research approach and be flexible about the methods and I suspect that the reason no other research of this kind has been undertaken with long-term survivors of adolescent cancer may be, in part, due to the evident challenges of devising a satisfactory research design and method.

Notes

1 Although Jamie was only 2 years post diagnosis he expressed a wish to participate, he had only received surgical treatment with no subsequent chemo or radiotherapy and, at his final follow-up appointment, regarded himself as a long-term survivor.
2 Phoebe was 2 years post diagnosis but had required only immediate surgery and clearly identified herself as a long-term survivor and wished to participate, therefore I have included her although she falls outside the criteria specified in Chapter 1.
3 The term 'adolescence and young adulthood' is used to cover the age range considered in this text. Where a distinction is necessary to differentiate the younger end of the continuum from the older, it will be specified in the discussion.
4 In no sense do I wish to suggest that experiencing cancer at other ages does not carry with it many difficulties and challenges, nor do I intend to diminish the needs of survivors of childhood cancer or the cancers of older adulthood. However, many of the needs of these other age groups are well researched and understood. Adolescents and young adults, on the cusp between childhood and adulthood, have only relatively recently come to be recognised as a group who can fall between services and whose needs have not been well understood in either the short term or the longer-term hence the importance of charting their long-term survivorship needs.
5 The theme of this chapter is the physical legacy of the cancer, thus it does by definition focus on late and long-term effects and physical symptoms that are experienced as negative. However, readers should be aware that this is a function of the topic of this chapter rather than a reflection of the tone taken by participants in relationship to surviving cancer. There are in this volume many extracts from survivors which are positive and reflect an optimistic approach and this chapter should be seen in the wider context of the other issues.

References

Albritton, K. and Bleyer, W.A. (2003) The Management of Cancer in the Older Adolescent, *European Journal of Cancer*, 39 (18): 2584–2599.

Appleby, J. and Deeming, C. (2001) Inverse Care Law, *Health Service Journal*, (111), 5760: 37, retrieved from: http://www.kingsfund.org.uk/publications/articles/ inverse_care_law.html, 22.6.08.

Apter, T. (2001) *The Myth of Maturity: what teenagers need from parents to become adults*, New York, W.W. Norton and Co Inc.

Arbuckle, J., Cotton, R., Eden, T.O.B., Jones, R. and Leonard, R. (2005) Who Should Care for Young People with Cancer? in Eden, T.O.B., Barr, R.D., Bleyer, A. and Whiteson, M. (eds) *Cancer and the Adolescent*, Oxford, Blackwell: 231–240.

Armstrong, L. with Jenkins, S. (2000) *It's Not About the Bike: my journey back to life*, New York, Putnam.

Aziz, N.M. (2007) Late Effects of Cancer Treatments, in Ganz, P.A. (ed.) *Cancer Survivorship: today and tomorrow*, New York, Springer: 54–76.

Barakat, L.P., Alderfer, M.A. and Kazak, A.E. (2006) Posttraumatic Growth in Adolescent Survivors of Cancer and their Mothers and Fathers, *Journal of Pediatric Psychology*, 31 (4): 413–419.

Birch, J.M. (2005) Patterns of Incidence of Cancer in Teenagers and Young Adults: Implications for Aetiology, in Eden, T.O.B., Barr, R.D., Bleyer, A. and Whiteson, M. (eds) *Cancer and the Adolescent*, Oxford, Blackwell: 13–31.

Birch, J.M., Pang, D., Alston, R.D., Rowan, S., Geraci, M., Moran, A. and Eden, T.O.B. (2008) Survival from Cancer in Teenagers and Young Adults in England 1979–2003, *British Journal of Cancer*, 99 (5): 830–835.

Broere, S. (2007) Sophie's Choice, *Contact*, Spring, Issue 34: 10.

Bryan, E. (2008) You Must Believe You Will Survive, *The Guardian*, 9 August.

Contact (2007) We made it Through … But will Never Forget Those that Didn't, *Contact*, Spring, 34: 5.

Cox, C.L., McLaughlin, R.A., Rai, S.N., Steen, B.D. and Hudson, M.M. (2005) Adolescent Survivors: a secondary analysis of a clinical trial targeting behaviour change, *Pediatric Blood Cancer*, 45 (2): 144–154.

Department of Health (2007) *Cancer Reform Strategy*, retrieved from: http://www.dh.gov.uk/en/Publicationsandstatistics/Publications/PublicationsPolicyAndGuidance/DH_081013, 3.09.08.

Drew, S. (2007) 'Having Cancer Changed my Life, and Changed my Life Forever': survival, illness legacy and service provision following cancer in childhood, *Chronic Illness*, 3 (4): 278–295.

Earle, C.C. (2007) Surveillance after Primary Therapy, in Ganz, P.A. (ed.) *Cancer Survivorship: today and tomorrow*, New York, Springer: 43–53.

Earle, C.C., Schrag, D., Woolf, S.H. and Ganz, P.A. (2007) The Survivorship Care Plan: what, why, how, and for whom, in Ganz, P.A. (ed.) *Cancer Survivorship: today and tomorrow*, New York, Springer: 287–293.

Eden, T. (2006) *Teenagers and Young Adults with Cancer 'The forgotten tribe'*, retrieved from: http://www.eolc-observatory.net/information/presentations/flash/teden_280606.swf, 7.7.06.

Eiser, C. (1998) Practitioner Review: long term consequences of childhood cancer, *Journal of Child Psychology and Psychiatry*, 39 (5): 621–633.

Feuerstein, M. (2007) Cancer Survivorship, Research, Practice and Policy, in Feuerstein, M. (ed.) *The Handbook of Cancer Survivorship*, New York, Springer: 483–494.

Field, D. (2002) Open Awareness and Dying: the use of denial and acceptance as coping strategies by hospice patients, *Nursing Times Research*, 7 (2): 118–127.

Fobair, P. (2007) Oncology Social Work for Survivorship, in Ganz, P.A. (ed.) *Cancer Survivorship: today and tomorrow*, New York, Springer: 14–27.

Frank, A. (2002) The Extrospection of Suffering: strategies of first-person illness narratives, in Patterson, W. (ed.) *Strategic Narrative: new perspectives on the power of personal and cultural stories*, Lanham, MD, Lexington Books: 165–177.

Gilbert, N. (2008) Research, Theory and Method, in Gilbert, N. (ed.) *Researching Social Life* (third edition), London, Sage: 21–40.

Glaser, B. and Strauss, A. (1967) *The Discovery of Grounded Theory*, Chicago, Aldine.

Grinyer A. (2007) *Young People Living with Cancer: implications for policy and practice*, Buckingham, Open University Press.

Grinyer, A. (2004) The Narrative Correspondence Method: what a follow-up study can tell us about the longer-term effect on participants in emotionally demanding research, *Qualitative Health Research*, 14 (10): 1326–1341.

Grinyer, A. (2002a) *Cancer in Young Adults: through parents' eyes*, Buckingham, Open University Press.

Grinyer, A. (2002b) The Anonymity of Research Participants: assumptions, ethics and practicalities, *Social Research Update*, Issue 36, University of Surrey.

Grinyer, A. and Thomas, C. (2001) Young Adults with Cancer: the effect on parents and families, *The International Journal of Palliative Nursing*, April 2001, 7 (4): 162–170.

Grbich, C. (1999) *Qualitative Research in Health*, London, Sage.

Hill, J.M., Kornblith, A.B., Jones, D., Freeman, A., Holland, J.F., Glicksman, A.S., Boyett, J.M., Lenherr, B., Brecher, M.L., Dubowy, R., Kung, F., Maurer, H. and Holland, J.C. (1998) A comparative study of the long term psychosocial functioning of childhood acute lymphoblastic leukaemia survivors treated by intrathecal methotrexate with or without cranial radiation, *Cancer*, 1 January, 82 (1): 201–218.

Hoffmann, B. (2007) The Employment and Insurance Concerns of Cancer Survivors, in Ganz, P.A. (ed.) *Cancer Survivorship: today and tomorrow*, New York, Springer: 272–282.

Hollen, P.J. and Hobbie W.L. (1993) Risk Taking and Decision Making of Adolescent Long Term Survivors of Cancer, *Oncology Nursing Forum*, June, 20 (5): 769–776.

Hollen, P.J., Hobbie, W.L. and Finley, S.M. (1999) Testing the Effects of a Decision

Making and Risk Reduction Program for Cancer-surviving Adolescents, *Oncology Nursing Forum*, October 26 (9): 1475–1486.

Hollen, P.J., Hobbie, W.L. and Finley, S.M. (1997) Cognitive Late Effect Factors Related to Decision Making and Risk Behaviors of Cancer-surviving Adolescents, *Cancer Nursing*, October 20 (5): 305–314.

Hollen, P.J., Hobbie, W.L., Finley, S.M. and Hiebert, S.M. (2001) The Relationship of Resiliency to Decision Making and Risk Behaviors of Cancer-surviving Adolescents, *Pediatric Oncology Nursing*, September–October, 18 (5): 188–204.

Jacobs, M. (1985) *The Presenting Past*, London, Harper and Row.

Jacobs, L.A., Alavi, J., DeMichele, A., Palmer, S., Stricker, C. and Vaughn, D. (2007) Comprehensive Long-term Follow-up, in Feuerstein, M. (ed.) *The Handbook of Cancer Survivorship*, New York, Springer: 397–415.

Keene, N., Hobbie, W. and Ruccione, K. (2000) *Childhood Cancer Survivors: a practical guide to your future*, Sebastopol, CA, O'Reilly.

Kelly, D. (2008), The Physical and Emotional Impact of Cancer in Adolescents and Young Adults, in Kelly, D. and Gibson, F. (eds) *Cancer Care for Adolescents and Young Adults*, Oxford, Blackwell: 23–43.

Kingma, A., Rammeloo, L.A., van der Does-van den Berg, A., Rekers-Mombarg, L. and Postma, A. (2000) Academic Career after Treatment for Acute Lymphoblastic Leukaemia, *Arch Dis Child*, May, 82 (5): 353–357.

Lahteenmaki, P.M., Holopainen, I., Krause, C.M., Heleius, H., Salmi, T.T. and Heikki, L.A. (2001) Cognitive Functions of Adolescent Childhood Cancer Survivors Assessed by Event-related Potentials, *Medical and Pediatric Oncology*, April, 36 (4): 442–450.

Langeveld, N. and Arbuckle, J. (2008) End of Treatment Issues: looking to the future, in Kelly, D. and Gibson, F. (eds) *Cancer Care for Adolescents and Young Adults*, Oxford, Blackwell: 147–162.

Levitt, G. and Eshelman, D. (2008) Long-term Effects of Cancer Treatment, in Kelly, D. and Gibson, F. (eds) *Cancer Care for Adolescents and Young Adults*, Oxford, Blackwell: 167–191.

Little, M., Sayers, E., Paul, K. and Jordens, C.F.C., (2000) On Surviving Cancer, *Journal of the Royal Society of Medicine*, October 2000, 93 (10): 501–503.

Mathieson, C.M. and Stam, H.J. (1995) Renegotiating Identity: cancer narratives, *Sociology of Health and Illness*, 17 (3): 283–306.

May, T. (1997) *Social Research: issues, methods and process*, Buckingham, Open University Press.

McKenzie, H. and Crouch, M. (2004) Discordant Feelings in the Lifeworld of Cancer Survivors, *Journal for the Social Study of Health, Illness and Medicine*, 8 (2): 139–157.

McQuellon, R.P. and Danhauer, S.C. (2007) Psychosocial Rehabilitation in Cancer Care, in Ganz, P.A. (ed.) *Cancer Survivorship: today and tomorrow*, New York, Springer: 238–250.

Mertens, A.C., Yasui, Y., Neglia, J.P., Potter, J.D., Nesbit, M.E. Jr., Ruccione, K., Smithson, W.A. and Robinson, L.L. (2001) Late [Morality] Experience in Five-year Survivors of Childhood and Adolescent Cancer: the Childhood Cancer Survivor Study, *Journal of Clinical Oncology*, July 1, 19 (13): 3163–3172.

Miedema, B., Hamilton, R. and Easley, J. (2007) From 'Invincibility' to 'Normalcy': Coping strategies of young adults during the cancer journey, *Palliative and Supportive Care*, 5, 41–49.

Miles, M.B. and Huberman, A.M. (1994) *Qualitative Data Analysis*, London, Sage.

Mor, V., Allen, S. and Malin, M. (1994) The Psychosocial Impact of Cancer on Older versus Younger Patients and their Families, *Cancer*, 74: 2118–2127.

Morgan, S. and Hubber, D. (2004) Setting up an Adolescent Service, in Gibson, F., Soanes, L. and Sepion, B. (eds) *Perspectives in Paediatric Oncology Nursing*, London, Whurr Publishers: 119–140.

Neville, K. (2007) Psychosocial Long Term Effects of Surviving Teenage Cancer, retrieved from http://www.nj.gov/health/ccr/documents/2005_1.pdf, 7.5.07.

Nezu, A.M. and Nezu, C.M. (2007) Psychological Distress, Depression, and Anxiety, in Feuerstein, M. (ed.), *The Handbook of Cancer Survivorship*, New York, Springer: 323–337.

Oeffinger, K.C. (2007) Book Review of *Cancer Survivorship: today and tomorrow*, (Ganz, P.A. ed. 2007), *The New England Journal of Medicine*, 357: 2209–2210.

Ozono, S., Saeki, T., Mantani, T., Ogata, A., Okamura, H. and Yamawaki, S. (2007) Factors Related to Posttraumatic Stress in Adolescent Survivors of Childhood Cancer and their Parents, *Supportive Care in Cancer*, 15 (3): 309–317.

Parsonnet, L. (2007) Psychosocial interventions with cancer survivors, retrieved from http://www.nj.gov/health/ccr/documents/2005_1.pdf, 7.5.07.

Parsons, T. (1951) *The Social System*, London, Routledge and Kegan Paul.

Phipps, S., Dunvant, M., Srivastava, D.K., Bowman, L. and Mulhern, R.K. (2000) Cognitive and Academic Functioning in Survivors of Pediatric Bone Marrow Transplantation, *Journal of Clinical Oncology*, March, 18 (5):1004–1011.

Prouty, D., Ward-Smith, P. and Hutto, C.J. (2006) The Lived Experiences of Adult Survivors of Childhood Cancer, *Journal of Pediaitric Oncology Nursing*, 23 (3) (May–June):143–151.

Reebals, J.F., Brown, R. and Buckner, E.B. (2006) Nurse Practice Issues Regarding Sperm Donation in Adolescent Male Cancer Patients, *Journal of Pediatric Oncology Nursing*, July–August, 23 (4): 182–188.

Reimers, T.S., Ehrenfels, S., Mortensen, E.L., Schmiegelow, M., Sonderkaer, S., Carstensen, H., Schmiegelow, K. and Muller, J. (2003) *Medical and Pediatric Oncology*, January, 40 (1): 26–34.

Robison, L.L. (2005) The Childhood Cancer Survivor Study: a resource for research of long-term outcomes among adult cancer survivors of childhood cancer, *Minnesota Medicine*, April, 88 (4): 45–49.

Robson, C. (1995) *Real World Research*, Oxford, Blackwell.

Schover, L.R. (2007) Reproductive Complications and Sexual Dysfunction in Cancer Survivors, in Ganz, P.A. (ed.) *Cancer Survivorship: today and tomorrow*, New York, Springer: 251–271.

Shaw, N., Wilford, H and Sepion, B. (2004) Semen Collection in Adolescents with Cancer, in Gibson, F., Soanes, L. and Sepion, B. (eds) *Perspectives in Paediatric Oncology Nursing*, London, Whurr Publishers: 141–157.

Silveri, M.M., Tzilos, G.K., Pimentel, P.J. and Yurgelun-Todd, D.A. (2004) Trajectories of Adolescent Emotional and Cognitive Development: effects of sex and risk for drug use, *Annals of the New York Academy of Science*, June, 1021: 363–370.

Soliman, H. and Agresta, S.V. (2008) Current Issues in Adolescent and Young Adult Cancer Survivorship, *Cancer Control*, 15 (1): 55–62.

Steinberg, S., Hartmann, R., Wisniewski, S., Berger, K., Beck, J.D. and Henze, G.

(1998) Late Sequelae of CNS Recurrence of Acute Lymphoblastic Leukemia in Childhood, *Klin Pediatr*, July–August, 210 (4): 200–206.

Stovall, E.L. (2007) Cancer Advocacy, in Ganz, P.A. (ed.) *Cancer Survivorship: today and tomorrow*, New York, Springer: 283–286.

The Children's Hospital of Philadelphia, Press Release (2006) Understanding the Late Effects of Childhood Cancer: 'A Mind–Body Approach' at the Children's Hospital of Philadelphia, retrieved from http://www.prnewswire.com/cgi-bin/micro_stories.pl?Tick=chop, 7.8.06.

Thomas, R. and Purdon, S. (1994) Telephone methods for social surveys, *Social Research Update*, 8, University of Surrey.

Tyc, V.L., Hadley, W. and Crockett, G. (2001) Prediction of health behaviours in pediatric cancer survivors, *Medical and Pediatric Oncology*, 2001, July, 37 (1): 42–46.

Van Dongen-Melman, J.E.W. (2000) Developing Psychosocial Aftercare for Children Surviving Cancer and their Families, *Acta Oncologica*, 39 (1): 23–31.

Wallace, W.H.B. and Brougham, M.F.H. (2005) Subfertility in Adolescents with Cancer: who is at risk and what can be done? in Eden, T.O.B., Barr, R.D., Bleyer, A. and Whiteson, M. (eds) *Cancer and the Adolescent*, Oxford, Blackwell: 133–154.

Wallace, W.H.B., Blacklay, A., Eiser, C., Davies, H., Hawkins, M., Levitt, G. and Jenney, M.E.M. (2001) Developing Strategies for Long term Follow-Up of Survivors of Childhood Cancer, *British Medical Journal*, 323: 271–274.

Wolff, S.N. (2007) The Burden of Cancer Survivorship, in Feuerstein, M. (ed.) *The Handbook of Cancer Survivorship*, New York, Springer: 7–18.

Zablotska, L.B., Matasar, M.J. and Neugut, A.I. (2007) Second Malignancies After Radiation Treatment and Chemotherapy for Primary Cancers, in Ganz, P.A. (ed.) *Cancer Survivorship: today and tomorrow*, New York, Springer: 225–237.

Zeltzer, L. (1993) Cancer in Adolescents and Young Adults Psychosocial Aspects: long-term survivors, *Cancer*, 71: 3463–3468.

Index

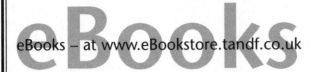